ANATOMY & PHYSIOLOGY
COLORING BOOK

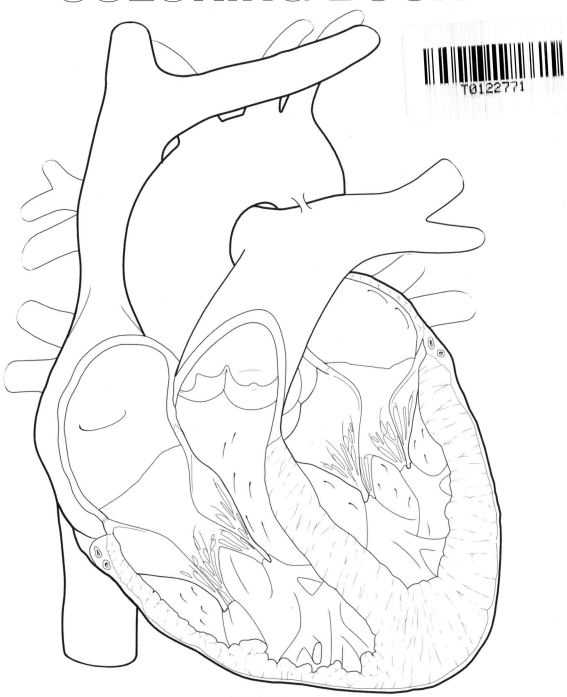

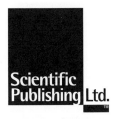

Scientific
Publishing Ltd.™

www.scientificpublishing.com

Dedicated to the special women in our life
Bonnie, Kristi, and Kay

©2024 Scientific Publishing Ltd. Elk Grove Village, IL USA

ISBN13: 978-1-935612-70-4

10 9 8 7 6 5 4 3

Item# SPL-CB

Published by Scientific Publishing Ltd.
167 Joey Drive, Elk Grove Village, IL 60007

Printed in China

Table of contents

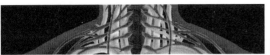

Introduction

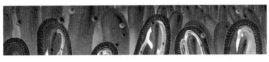

Cells & Tissues

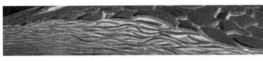

The Integumentary System

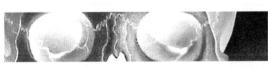

The Skeletal System

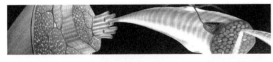

The Muscular System

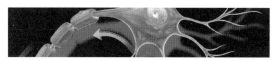

The Nervous System

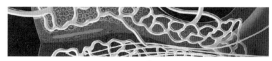

The Endocrine System

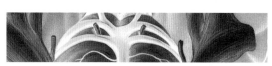

The Vascular System

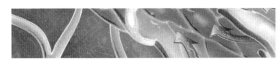

The Lymphatic System

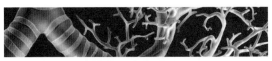

The Respiratory System

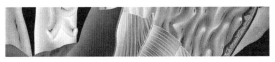

The Digestive System

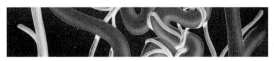

The Urinary System

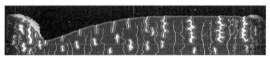

The Reproductive System

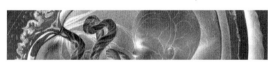

Pregnancy & Birth

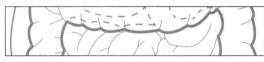

Anatomical glossary

Using this book

Our coloring book is organized by systems of the body. The line drawings and supporting text can help break down complex anatomical topics. The physiology areas graphically explain the processes of the functioning of human beings. The activity of coloring the labeled images can enhance the learning experience.

Anatomical and physiological items to be colored are indicated by an open bullet (○) and a number, followed by the name or definition. The specific color selected should match the numbered area or definition on the illustration. When multiple images of the same subject are on the same page we suggest the same color be used to indicate similar parts. Anatomical and physiological items indicated with a dash (–) should not be colored. These items are used to signify supportive anatomy or areas of reference.

We suggest using good quality colored pencils, preferably a boxed set of 24 or larger. Colored pencils will provide better definition and flexibility because they can be used for shading. Colored pencils can also be blended to provide an even wider range of color selections. The use of markers can cause the ink to bleed through the paper and transfer to the underlying sheet.

Colors affect us both psychologically and perceptually by helping us determine how objects appear positioned next to another. Cool colors (blue, green and violet) seem to appear farther from the observer or recede. Warm colors (red, yellow and orange) appear to advance or come forward in a picture. Neutral colors include black, white, gray, tans and browns. They're commonly combined with brighter accent colors but they can also be used on their own. The meanings and impressions of neutral colors depend more on the colors around them. Shades are made by mixing a pure color with black. Tints are made by mixing a pure color with white. We recommend the largest areas be colored the lightest and smaller areas have the highest color contrast.

The pages in the book are perforated near the spine and can be removed for individual study or to make coloring easier. At the end of the book you will find an abridged glossary to help in your studies and general understanding of anatomical/physiological terms.

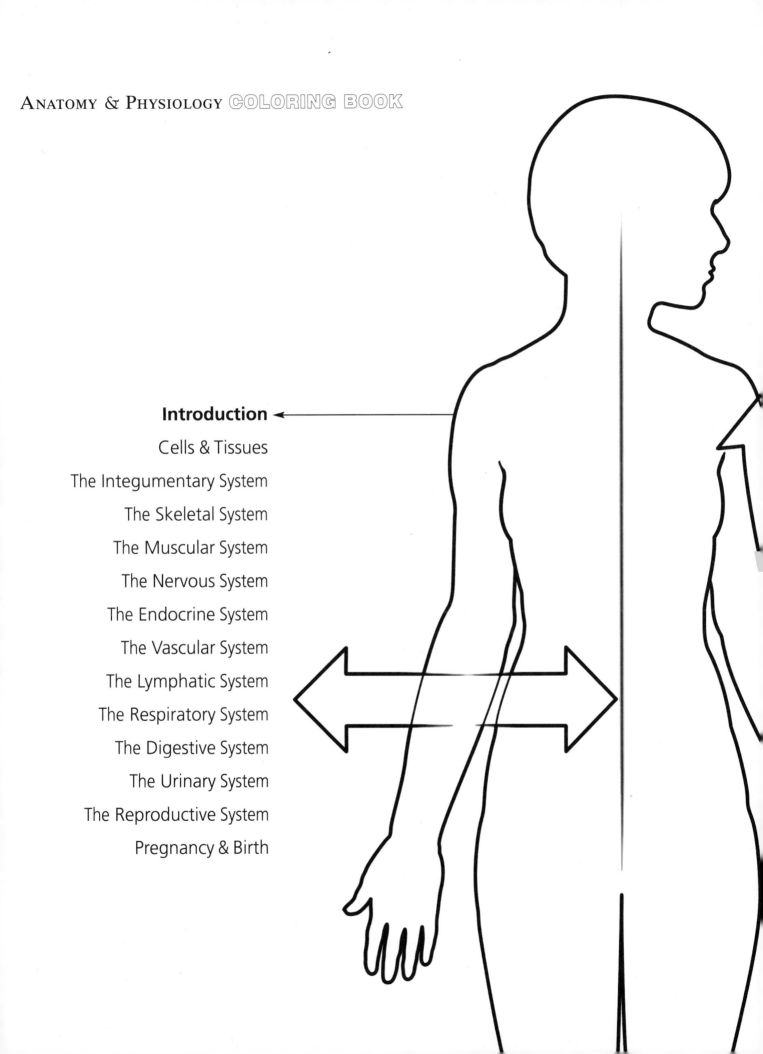

ANATOMY & PHYSIOLOGY COLORING BOOK

Introduction

Systems of the human body

As humans, our bodies need to be able to grow, to move and to repair as necessary. We need to be able to sense our environment and to respond appropriately. We depend on the air we breathe and the food we eat to give us energy. As organisms, we need to be able to reproduce. We have specialized systems to handle these functions, including an internal transportation system (*vascular*) connecting the systems.

The Integumentary System
The integuement system includes the skin and associated glands, hair and nails.

The Muscular System
The muscular system interacts with the skeletal system to allow us to produce a wide variety of motions.

The Skeletal System
The skeletal system provides structure and support, forming the framework for the body.

The Nervous System
The nervous system is composed of two integrated subdivisions (*CNS and PNS*) that are responsible for conducting and processing sensory and motor information.

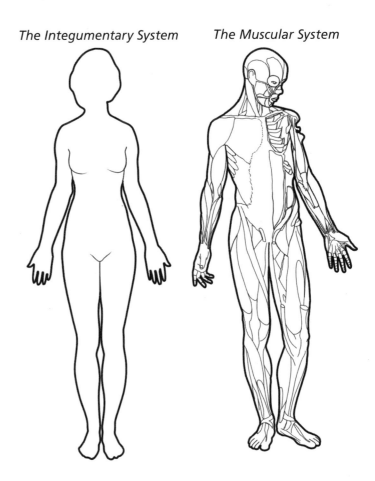

The Integumentary System   *The Muscular System*

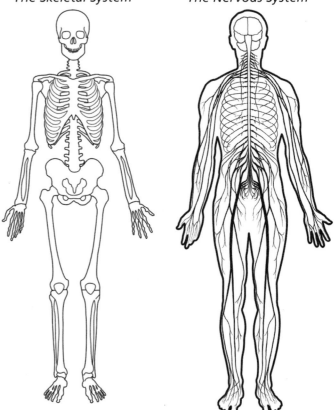

The Skeletal System   *The Nervous System*

Systems of the human body

The Endocrine System
The endocrine system is made up of organs and glands that produce hormones and internal chemical messengers that regulate and control functions within the body.

The Vascular System
Nutrients are delivered and waste products are removed from the body through the heart, blood vessels and blood of the vascular system.

The Endocrine System   *The Vascular System*

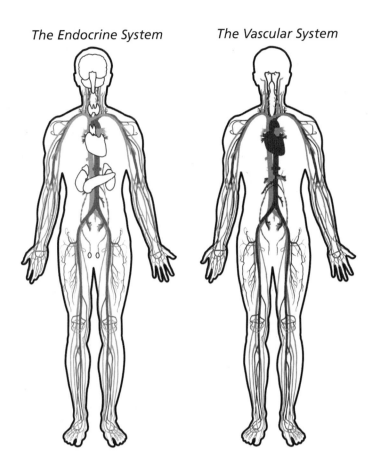

The Lymphatic System
The lymphatic system is an extensive network of vessels and nodes that forms a central part of the body's defenses against illness and injury.

The Respiratory System
The respiratory system provides the means to exchange oxygen and carbon dioxide at the cellular level.

The Lymphatic System   *The Respiratory System*

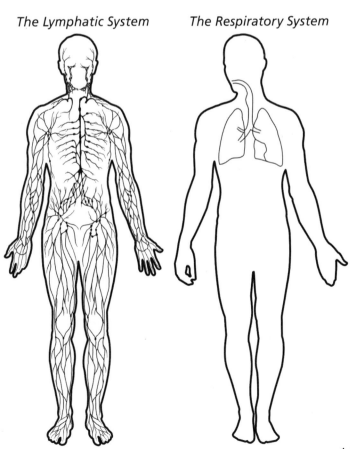

Systems of the human body

The Digestive System

The Urinary System

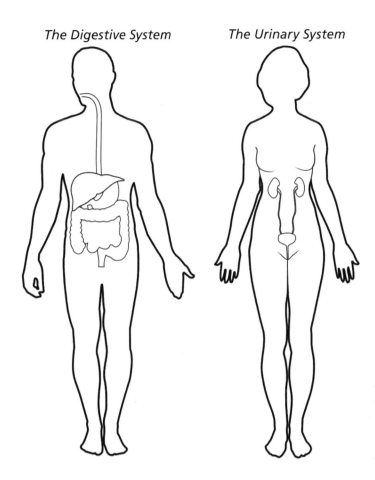

The Digestive System
The digestive system, or gastrointestinal tract, is essentially a muscular tube in which intake, digestion and absorption of nutrients take place.

The Urinary System
The urinary system is responsible for three major functions in the body: removing wastes, maintaining normal water volume, and controlling acid-base balance in the bloodstream.

The Reproductive System

Pregnancy and Birth

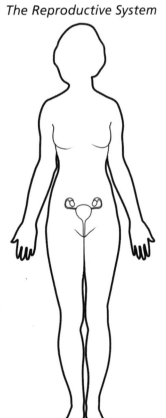

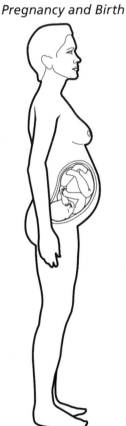

The Reproductive System
Humans reproduce by sexual reproduction involving male and female reproductive cells (*sperm and ova*).

Pregnancy and Birth
Pregnancy lasts approximately 40 weeks from the first day of the last menstrual period.

Organizational levels

Systems are made up of organs and specialized tissues and cells. An example of the system level of organization is the cardiovascular system, which includes the heart, the circulatory system (*a network of blood vessels*), and blood. Organs, such as the small intestine, are composed of several types of tissues, each with a specific function. Tissues are made up of groups of cells carrying out a common purpose. Cells are the smallest functional and structural components of the body.

System level
Digestive system

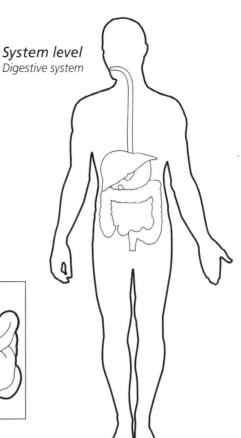

Cellular level
Ciliated columnar epithelium

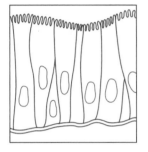

Tissue level
Intestinal lining

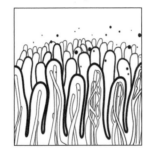

Organ level
Small intestine

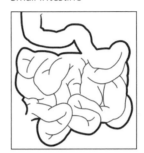

Anatomical terms

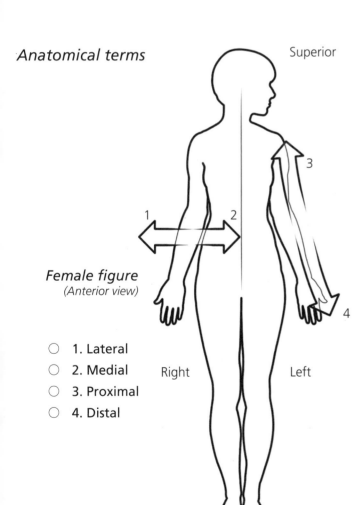

Superior

Right   Left

Inferior

Female figure
(Anterior view)

○ 1. Lateral
○ 2. Medial
○ 3. Proximal
○ 4. Distal

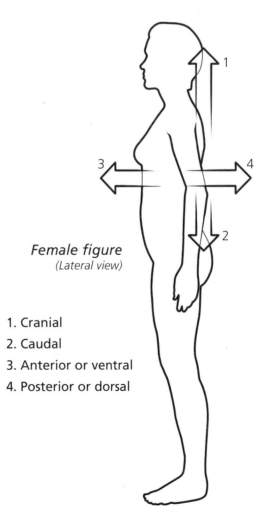

Female figure
(Lateral view)

○ 1. Cranial
○ 2. Caudal
○ 3. Anterior or ventral
○ 4. Posterior or dorsal

1.4

Anatomical terms

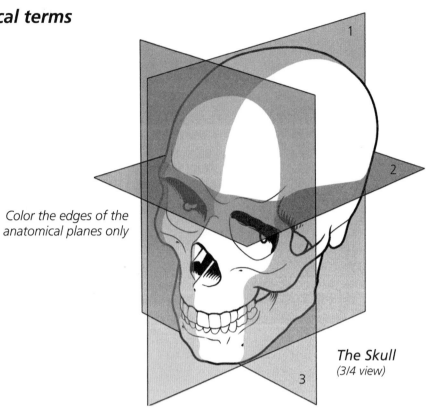

Color the edges of the anatomical planes only

Anatomical planes

○ 1. Sagittal
○ 2. Transverse
○ 3. Coronal

The Skull
(3/4 view)

Anatomical planes: 1

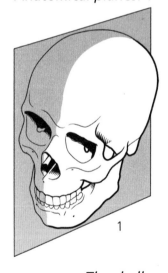

Anatomical planes: 2

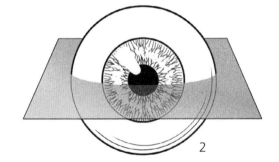

Anatomical planes: 3

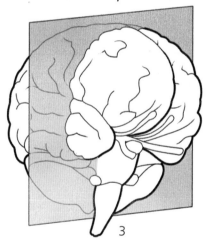

The skull
(1 view)

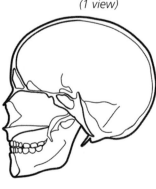

The eye
(2 view)

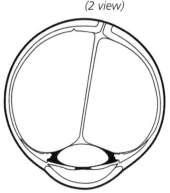

The brain
(3 view)

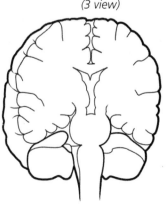

1.5

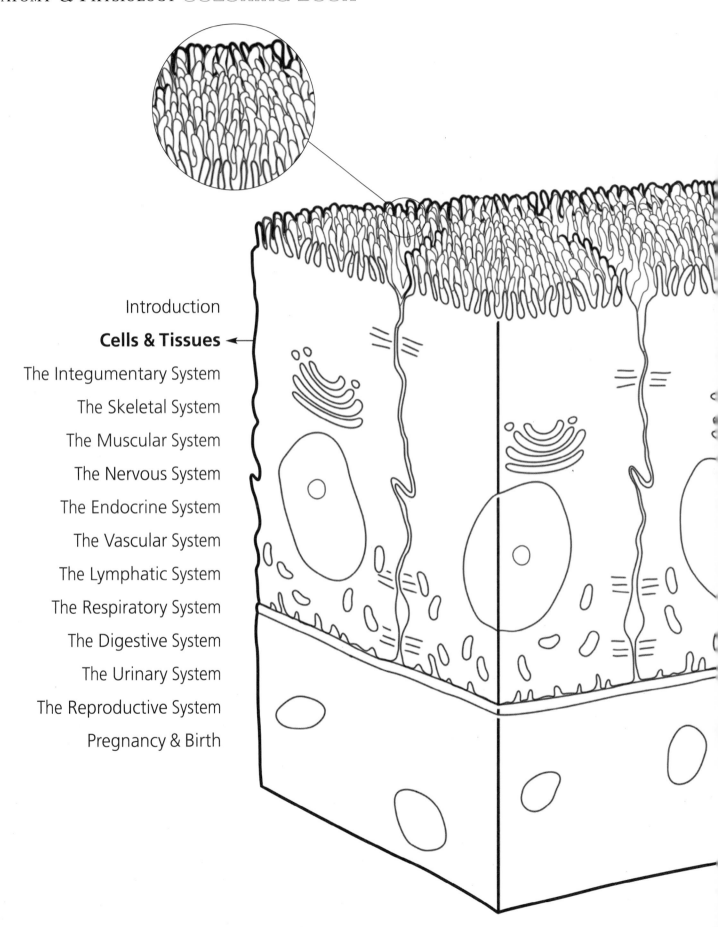

ANATOMY & PHYSIOLOGY COLORING BOOK

The cell

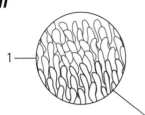

The human body contains trillions of cells, the smallest functional and structural components of the body. Cells vary in size, shape and purpose, from the red blood cell, carrying oxygen throughout the body, to the neuron, a unit of the nervous system. Different kinds of cells combine to form tissues, groups of cells working together to perform a specific function.

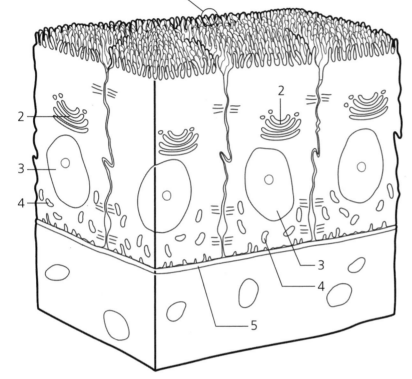

Type Columnar
Location lining of large bronchioles (respiratory)

○ 1. Microvilli
○ 2. Golgi apparatus
○ 3. Nucleus
○ 4. Mitochondria
○ 5. Basement membrane

> **Coloring guide suggestion**
> *When coloring, use same color to indicate similar parts*

Tissues

Epithelial tissue: Simple

Type: Squamous
Location: Alveoli (*respiratory*)

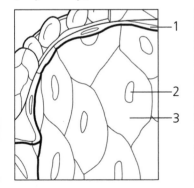

○ 1. Basement membrane
○ 2. Nucleus
○ 3. Cell body

Type: Cuboidal
Location: Distal convoluted tubule (*kidney*)

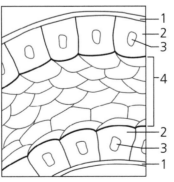

○ 1. Basement membrane
○ 2. Cell body
○ 3. Nucleus
○ 4. Tubule lumen

Type: Columnar
Location: Lining of GI tract (*digestive*)

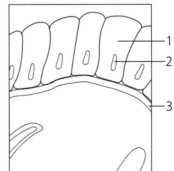

○ 1. Cell body
○ 2. Nucleus
○ 3. Basement membrane

Type: Columnar (*ciliated*)
Location: Lining of large bronchioles (*respiratory*)

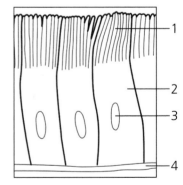

○ 1. Cilia
○ 2. Cell body
○ 3. Nucleus
○ 4. Basement membrane

Coloring guide suggestion
When coloring, use same color to indicate similar parts

Tissues

Epithelial tissue: Stratified

Type: Stratified squamous
Location: Esophageal lining

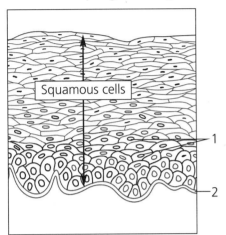

Squamous cells

○ 1. Nuclei
○ 2. Basement membrane

Epithelial tissue: Glandular

Type: Exocrine
Location: Goblet cells (*respiratory*)

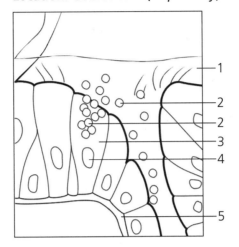

○ 1. Mucus
○ 2. Secretory vesicle
○ 3. Cell body
○ 4. Nucleus
○ 5. Basement membrane

Type: Exocrine
Location: Sebaceous gland (*skin*)

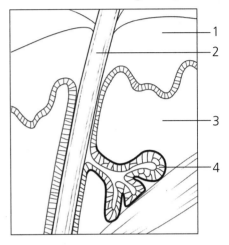

○ 1. Epidermis
○ 2. Hair shaft
○ 3. Dermis
○ 4. Sebaceous gland

Muscle tissue

Type: Skeletal
Location: Voluntary muscles

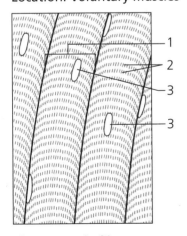

○ 1. Muscle fiber
− 2. Striations
○ 3. Nucleus

Type: Cardiac
Location: Heart

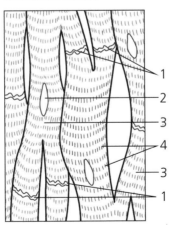

○ 1. Intercalated discs
○ 2. Nucleus
○ 3. Cardiac muscle cell
− 4. Striations

Type: Smooth
Location: Digestive organs

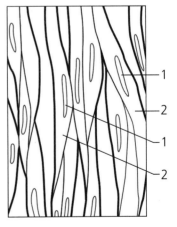

○ 1. Nucleus
○ 2. Smooth muscle cell

Tissues

Connective tissue proper: *Loose*

Type: Areolar
Location: Fascia

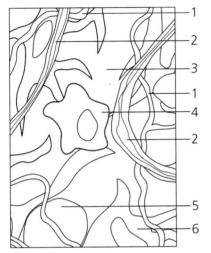

○ 1. Elastic fiber
○ 2. Collagen fiber
○ 3. Ground substance
○ 4. Macrophage
○ 5. Adipocyte
○ 6. Fibroblast

Type: Adipose
Location: Subcutaneous layer (*skin*)

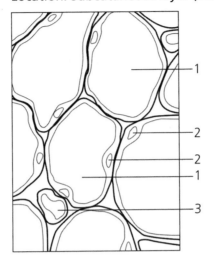

○ 1. Adipocyte
○ 2. Nucleus
○ 3. Blood vessel

Type: Reticular
Location: Spleen

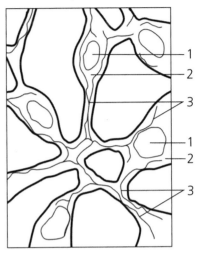

○ 1. Nucleus
○ 2. Cell body
– 3. Recticular fibers

Connective tissue proper: *Dense*

Type: Regular
Location: Tendons, ligaments

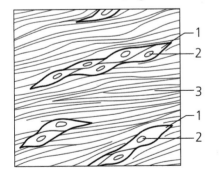

○ 1. Fibroblast
○ 2. Nucleus
○ 3. Collagen fibers

Type: Irregular
Location: Dermis, joint capsules

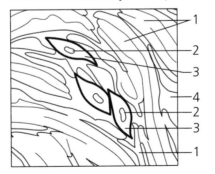

○ 1. Collagen fibers
○ 2. Nucleus
○ 3. Fibroblast
○ 4. Ground substance

Type: Elastic
Location: Around arteries

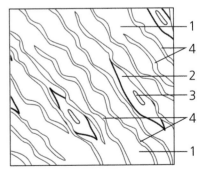

○ 1. Ground substance
○ 2. Fibroblast
○ 3. Nucleus
○ 4. Elastic fibers

Tissues

Supporting tissue

Type: Hyaline cartilage
Location: Larynx, trachea, end of long bones

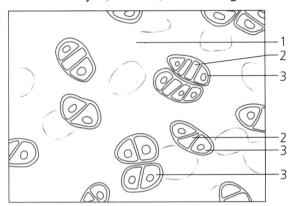

○ 1. Matrix

○ 2. Lacuna

○ 3. Chondrocyte

Type: Elastic cartilage
Location: External ear

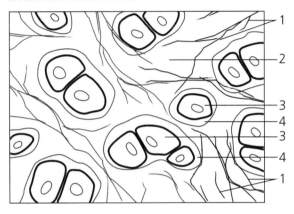

— 1. Elastic fibers in matrix

○ 2. Matrix

○ 3. Chondrocyte

○ 4. Lacuna

Type: Fibrocartilage
Location: Intervertebral discs

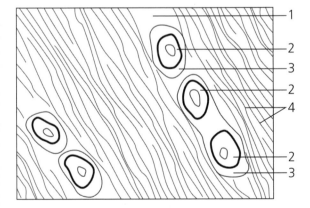

○ 1. Matrix

○ 2. Chondrocyte

○ 3. Lacuna

— 4. Collagen fibers in matrix

Type: Bone

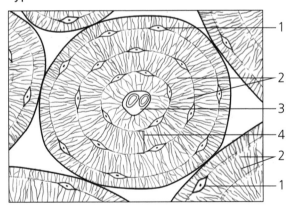

○ 1. Osteocyte

— 2. Canaliculi

○ 3. Central canal with artery, vein and nerve

○ 4. Lamella (*layers*)

2.4

Tissues

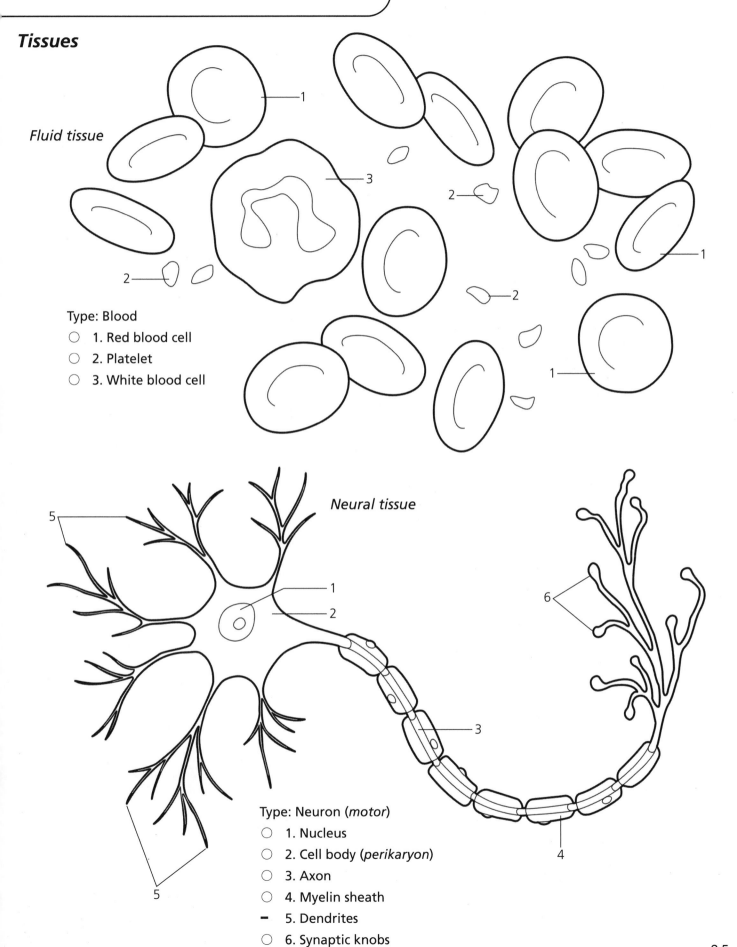

Fluid tissue

Type: Blood

○ 1. Red blood cell

○ 2. Platelet

○ 3. White blood cell

Neural tissue

Type: Neuron (*motor*)

○ 1. Nucleus

○ 2. Cell body (*perikaryon*)

○ 3. Axon

○ 4. Myelin sheath

– 5. Dendrites

○ 6. Synaptic knobs

ANATOMY & PHYSIOLOGY COLORING BOOK

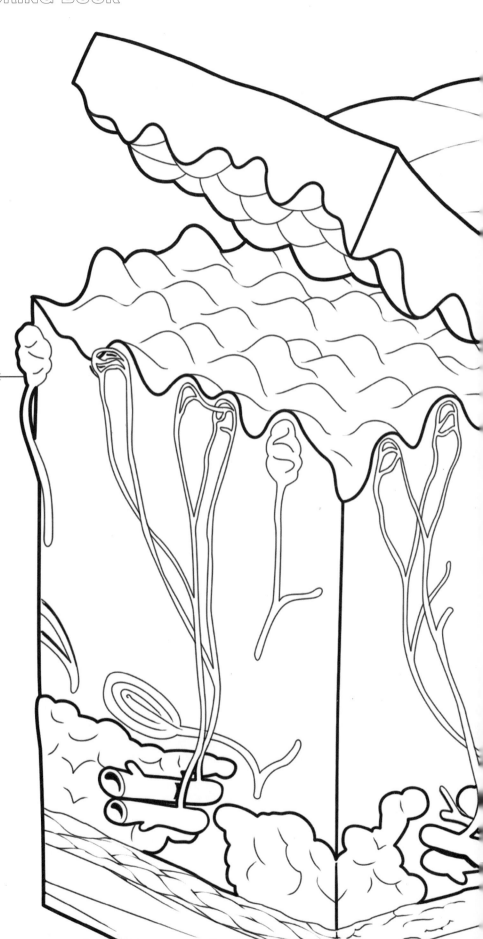

The INTEGUMENTARY System

Inside the skin

The integumentary system includes the skin and associated glands, hair and nails. The skin is a highly elastic organ covering the entire outer surface of the body. It performs numerous functions essential to survival, including: prevention of fluid loss from body tissues, protection against environmental toxins and microorganisms, reception of heat, cold and pain sensations, regulation of normal body temperature and maintenance of calcium levels.

Thick skin
Hairless

Thin skin

- 1. Opening of sweat duct
- ○ 2. Friction ridges
- ○ 3. Epidermis

Coloring guide suggestion
When coloring, use same color to indicate similar parts

- ○ 1. Epidermis ⟷
- ○ 2. Dermis ⟷
- ○ 3. Hypodermis (subcutaneous layer) ⟶
- ○ 4. Sweat gland pore
- ○ 5. Merkel cell
- ○ 6. Vascular plexus
- ○ 7. Free nerve endings
- ○ 8. Ruffini's corpuscle
- ○ 9. Sweat gland
- ○ 10. Arteriole
- ○ 11. Venule
- ○ 12. Sensory nerve
- ○ 13. Adipose tissue
- ○ 14. Muscle
- ○ 15. Connective fibrous tissue

3.1

The INTEGUMENTARY System

Inside the skin

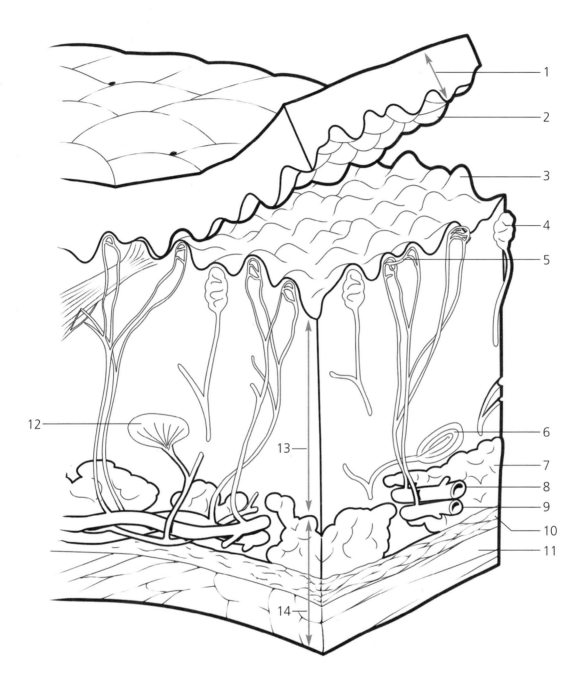

○ 1. Epidermis ←→
○ 2. Epidermal ridges
○ 3. Dermal papillae
○ 4. Meissner's corpuscle
○ 5. Vascular plexus
○ 6. Lamellated corpuscle
○ 7. Adipose tissue
○ 8. Arteriole
○ 9. Venule
○ 10. Connective fibrous tissue
○ 11. Muscle
○ 12. Ruffini's corpuscle
○ 13. Dermis ←→
○ 14. Hypodermis (*subcutaneous*) ←→

The INTEGUMENTARY System

Accessory structures

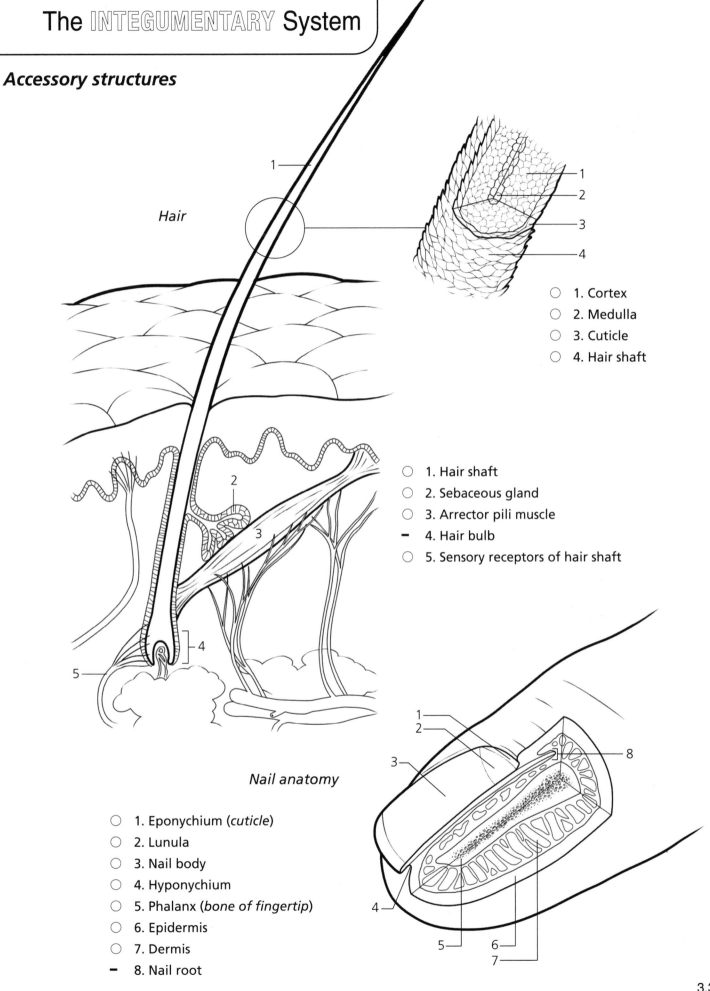

Hair

○ 1. Cortex
○ 2. Medulla
○ 3. Cuticle
○ 4. Hair shaft

○ 1. Hair shaft
○ 2. Sebaceous gland
○ 3. Arrector pili muscle
– 4. Hair bulb
○ 5. Sensory receptors of hair shaft

Nail anatomy

○ 1. Eponychium (*cuticle*)
○ 2. Lunula
○ 3. Nail body
○ 4. Hyponychium
○ 5. Phalanx (*bone of fingertip*)
○ 6. Epidermis
○ 7. Dermis
– 8. Nail root

3.3

The INTEGUMENTARY System

Epidermal layers

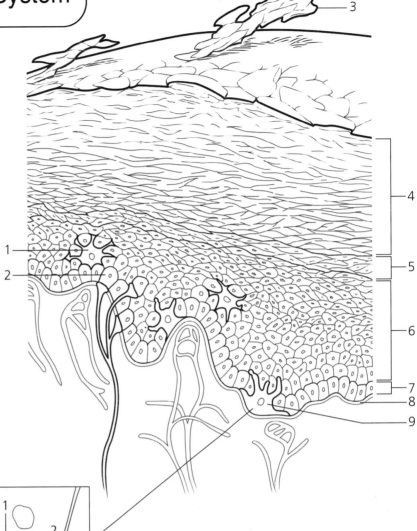

- ○ 1. Dendritic (*Langerhans*) cells
- ○ 2. Merkel (*tactile*) cells
- ○ 3. Sloughing keratinocytes
- ○ 4. Stratum corneum*
- ○ 5. Stratum granulosum
- ○ 6. Stratum spinosum
- ○ 7. Stratum basale
- ○ 8. Basement membrane
- ○ 9. Melanocyte

*Stratum corneum
[between the stratum granulosum and the stratum lucidum in thick skin only]

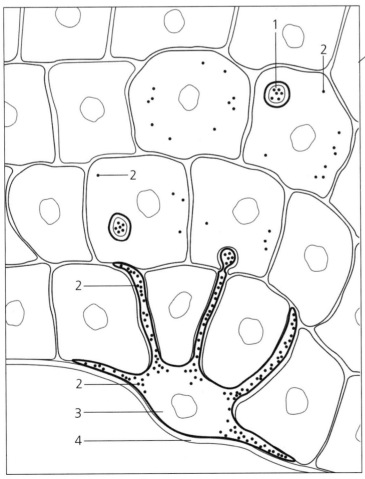

Skin color

Skin gets its color primarily from melanin, a brown pigment produced by the melanocytes in the epidermis. Individual skin color can range from pale yellow to black, depending on the amount of melanin the melanocytes produce. In some fair-skinned people, uneven distribution of melanocytes results in spots of pigmentation called freckles. More melanin is produced when the skin is exposed to sunlight, creating a darker skin tone or tan to help protect against UV radiation.

- ○ 1. Melanosome
- – 2. Melanin
- ○ 3. Melanocyte
- ○ 4. Basement membrane

Skin sensors

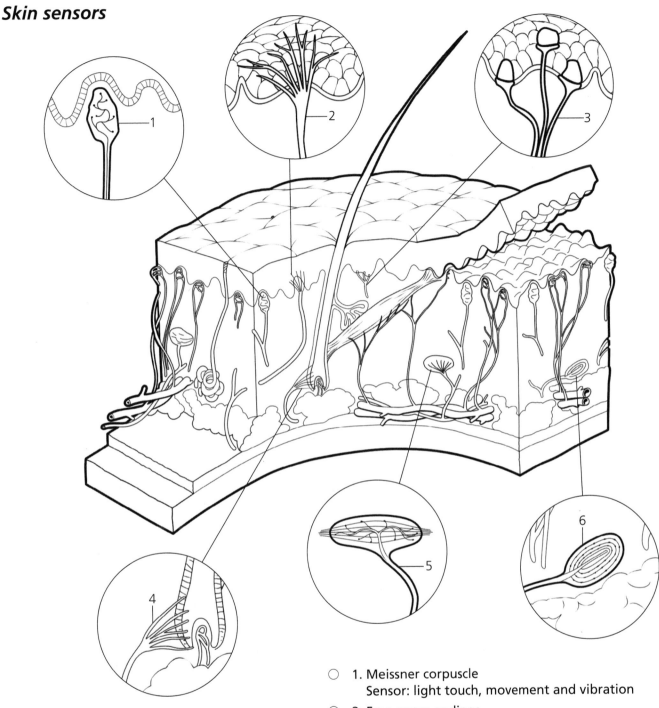

Our ability to sense and respond to the environment includes sensation, the awareness of a stimulus, and perception, the understanding of the meaning of a stimulus. Sensory receptors, highly specialized nerve cells, help us detect light, temperature and other kinds of energy. These receptors transduce, or convert, the various types of energy into signals understood by the nervous system. Each type of receptor responds to a specific form of energy–rods and cones respond to light, and olfactory receptor cells respond to odorants (chemicals).

○ 1. Meissner corpuscle
   Sensor: light touch, movement and vibration

○ 2. Free nerve endings
   Sensor: temperature, pressure and pain

○ 3. Merkel cell
   Sensor: light touch

○ 4. Sensory receptors of hair shaft
   Sensor: distortion and movement across the body surface

○ 5. Ruffini corpuscle
   Sensor: tension, pressure and skin distortion

○ 6. Pacinian (*lamellated*) corpuscle
   Sensor: heavy pressure and vibration

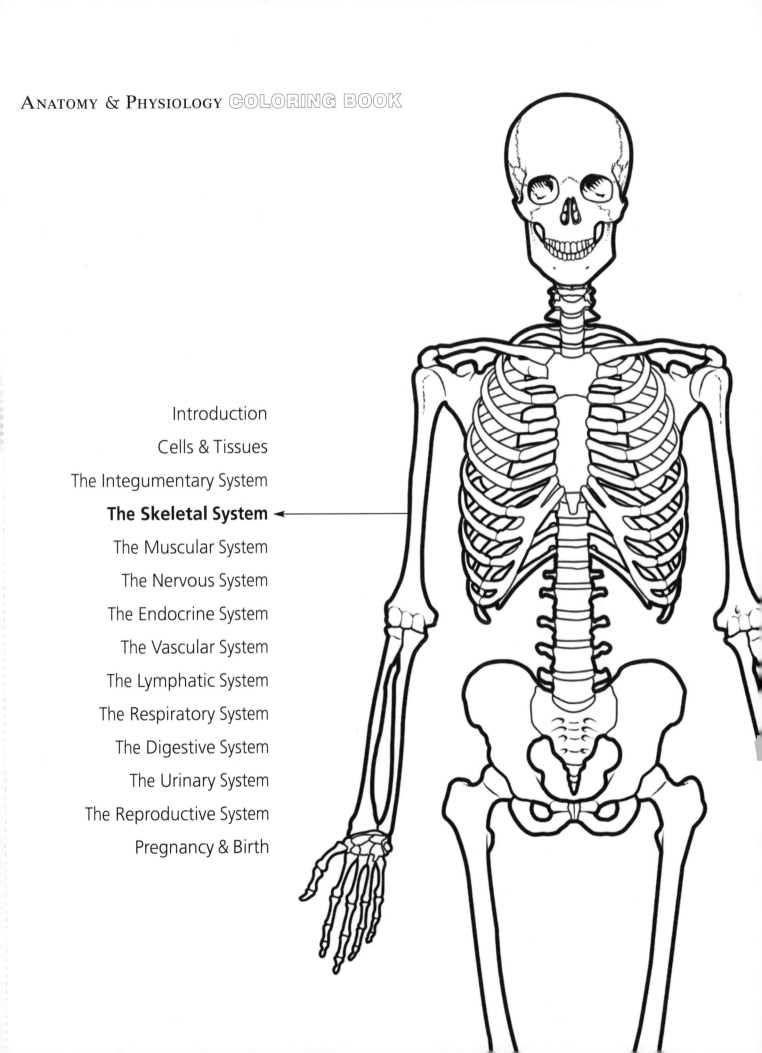

ANATOMY & PHYSIOLOGY COLORING BOOK

The SKELETAL System

System overview

The skeletal system provides structure and support, forming the framework for the body. The skeleton works together with the muscular system to allow a wide variety of motions, including standing, sitting and movement of body parts. In addition to providing support and structure, the skeletal system has several other functions. Bones store minerals, especially calcium, and lipids (in the yellow bone marrow) as reserves. Red bone marrow is the primary site for hemopoiesis, or blood cell formation.

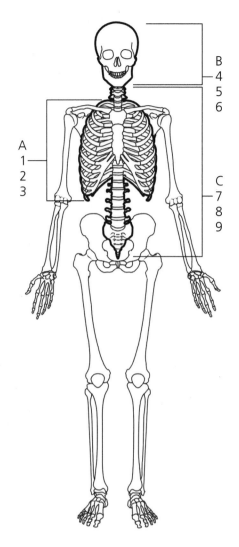

The axial skeleton

A – Thoracic cage
1. Sternum
2. Ribs
3. Thoracic vertebrae

B – Skull and associated bones
4. Skull
5. Auditory ossicles
6. Hyoid

C – Vertebral column
7. Vertebrae
8. Sacrum
9. Coccyx

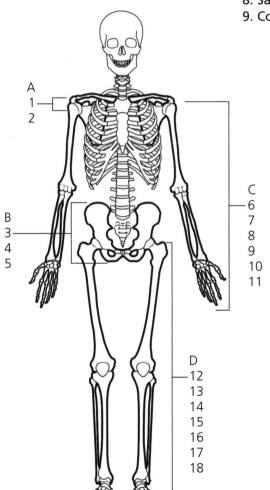

The appendicular skeleton

A – Pectoral girdles
1. Clavicle
2. Scapula

B – Pelvic girdle
3. Ossa coxae (2)
4. Sacrum
5. Coccyx

C – Upper limbs
6. Humerus
7. Radius
8. Ulna
9. Carpal bones
10. Metacarpal bones
11. Phalanges

D – Lower limbs
12. Femur
13. Patella
14. Tibia
15. Fibula
16. Tarsal bones
17. Metatarsal bones
18. Phalanges

The SKELETAL System

Bone structure

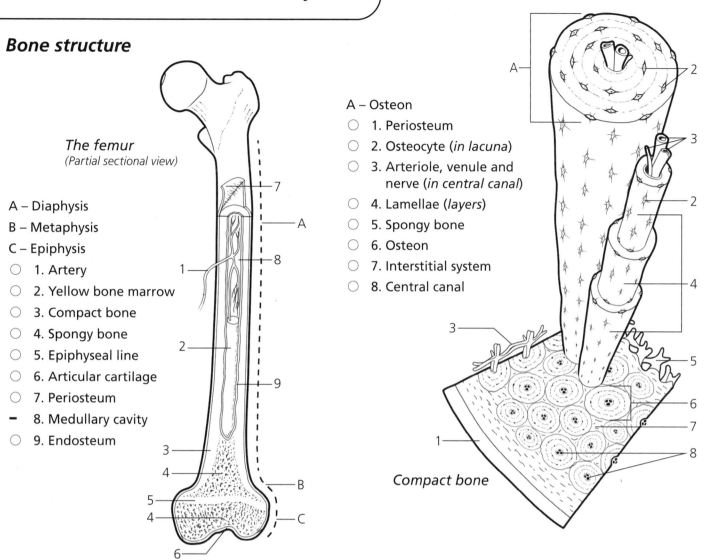

The femur
(Partial sectional view)

A – Diaphysis
B – Metaphysis
C – Epiphysis
○ 1. Artery
○ 2. Yellow bone marrow
○ 3. Compact bone
○ 4. Spongy bone
○ 5. Epiphyseal line
○ 6. Articular cartilage
○ 7. Periosteum
– 8. Medullary cavity
○ 9. Endosteum

A – Osteon
○ 1. Periosteum
○ 2. Osteocyte (*in lacuna*)
○ 3. Arteriole, venule and nerve (*in central canal*)
○ 4. Lamellae (*layers*)
○ 5. Spongy bone
○ 6. Osteon
○ 7. Interstitial system
○ 8. Central canal

Compact bone

PHYSIOLOGY:
Bone remodeling cycle

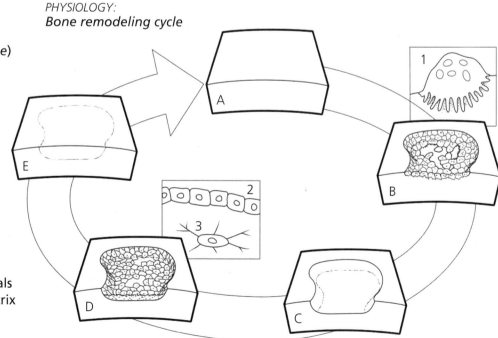

A – The cycle begins on the trabecular plates (*mature bone*)

B – Activation of dormant cells (osteoclast precursors) into bone break down cells called
  ○ 1. Osteoclast

C – Osteoclasts dissolve old bone and dig microscopic cavities

D – Bone-forming osteoblasts are attracted to the cavities and begin filling them with a collagen matrix
  ○ 2. Osteoblasts
  ○ 3. Osteocyte

E – Calcium and phosphorus crystals are added to the collagen matrix to strengthen and harden the bone

The SKELETAL System

The skeleton

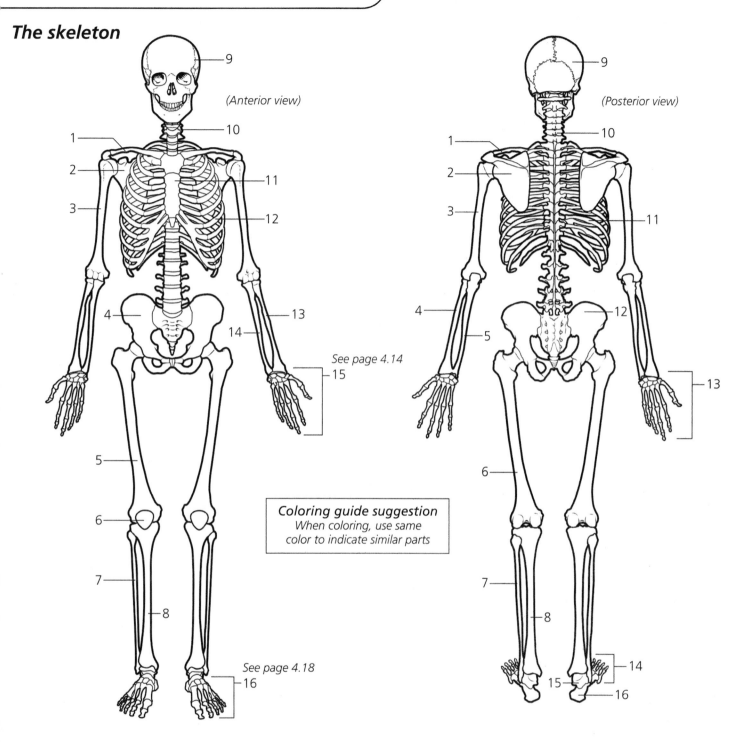

(Anterior view)

(Posterior view)

Coloring guide suggestion
When coloring, use same
color to indicate similar parts

See page 4.14

See page 4.18

○ 1. Clavicle
○ 2. Scapula
○ 3. Humerus
○ 4. Os coxae
    Ilium, Pubis, Ischium
○ 5. Femur
○ 6. Patella
○ 7. Fibula
○ 8. Tibia

○ 9. Skull
○ 10. Vertebral column
○ 11. Sternum
○ 12. Ribs
○ 13. Radius
○ 14. Ulna
○ 15. Bones of the hand
○ 16. Bones of the feet

○ 1. Clavicle
○ 2. Scapula
○ 3. Humerus
○ 4. Radius
○ 5. Ulna
○ 6. Femur
○ 7. Fibula
○ 8. Tibia
○ 9. Skull

○ 10. Vertebral column
○ 11. Ribs
○ 12. Os coxae
    Ilium, Pubis, Ischium
○ 13. Bones of the hand
○ 14. Bones of the feet
○ 15. Talus
○ 16. Calcaneus

The SKELETAL System

Axial skeleton

The skull
(Anterior view)

○ 1. Parietal bone
○ 2. Sphenoid bone
○ 3. Temporal bone
○ 4. Ethmoid bone
○ 5. Lacrimal bone
○ 6. Nasal bone
– 7. Infra orbital foramen
○ 8. Vomer
○ 9. Maxilla
○ 10. Mandible
– 11. Mental foramen
○ 12. Frontal bone
– 13. Orbit
○ 14. Zygomatic bone
– 15. Teeth

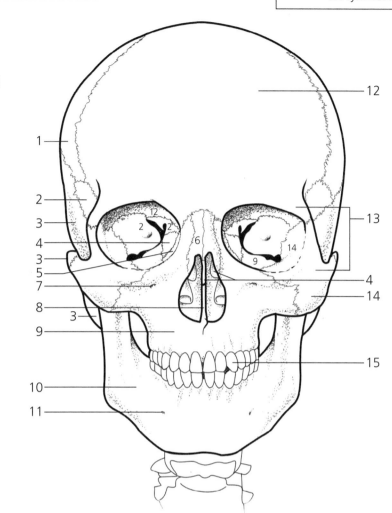

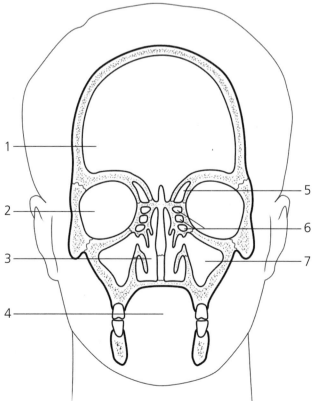

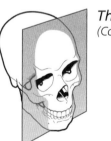

The skull
(Coronal section)

○ 1. Cranial cavity
○ 2. Orbit
– 3. Nasal cavity
– 4. Oral cavity
○ 5. Frontal sinus
○ 6. Ethmoid sinuses
○ 7. Maxillary sinus

4.4

The SKELETAL System

Axial skeleton

The skull
(Lateral view)

- ○ 1. Frontal bone
- ○ 2. Nasal bone
- ○ 3. Zygomatic bone
- − 4. Infra orbital foramen
- ○ 5. Maxilla
- − 6. Teeth
- ○ 7. Mandible
- − 8. Mental foramen
- ○ 9. Parietal bone
- ○ 10. Sphenoid bone
- ○ 11. Temporal bone
- ○ 12. Occipital bone
- − 13. External auditory canal
- − 14. Mastoid process
- ○ 15. Styloid process

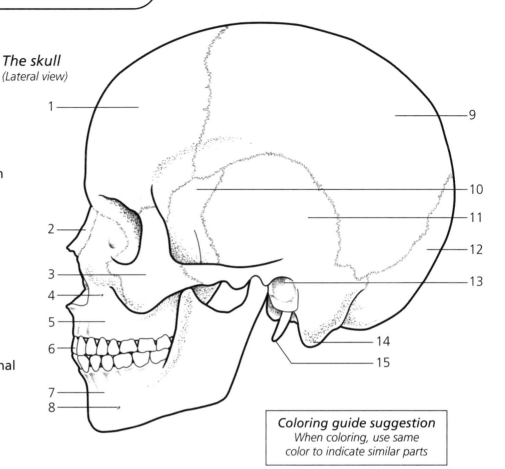

Coloring guide suggestion
When coloring, use same color to indicate similar parts

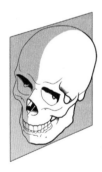

The skull
(Sagittal section)

- ○ 1. Frontal bone
- ○ 2. Frontal sinus
- ○ 3. Ethmoid sinuses
- ○ 4. Nasal bone
- ○ 5. Sphenoid sinus
- ○ 6. Maxilla
- − 7. Teeth
- ○ 8. Mandible
- ○ 9. Parietal bone
- ○ 10. Sphenoid bone
- ○ 11. Occipital bone
- ○ 12. Temporal bone
- ○ 13. Ethmoid bone
- ○ 14. Vomer
- ○ 15. Styloid process

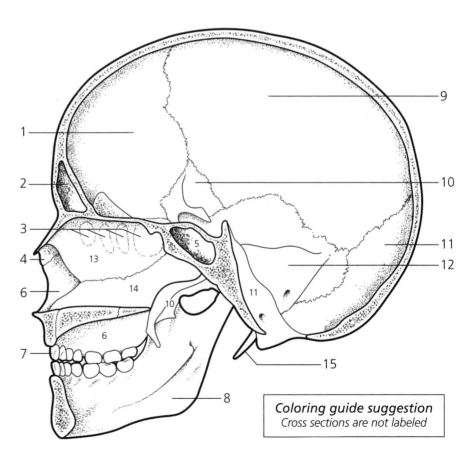

Coloring guide suggestion
Cross sections are not labeled

4.5

The SKELETAL System

Axial skeleton

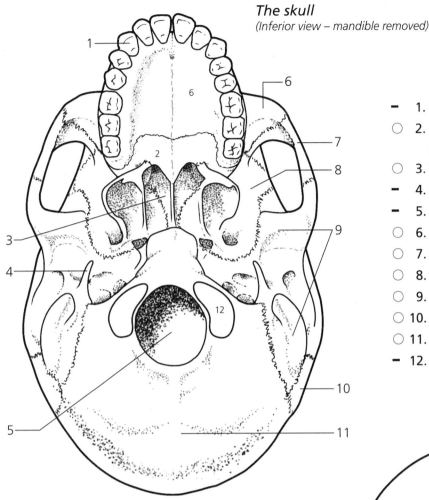

The skull
(Inferior view – mandible removed)

- 1. Teeth
- ○ 2. Palatine bone (*horizontal plate*)
- ○ 3. Vomer
- 4. Styloid process
- 5. Foramen magnum
- ○ 6. Maxilla (*upper jaw*)
- ○ 7. Zygomatic bone
- ○ 8. Sphenoid bone
- ○ 9. Temporal bone
- ○ 10. Parietal bone
- ○ 11. Occipital bone
- 12. Occipital condyle

The skull
(3/4 view)

Cranial sutures (selected)

- ○ 1. Squamous s.
- ○ 2. Sphenofrontal s.
- ○ 3. Sphenosquamous s.
- ○ 4. Frontozygomatic s.
- ○ 5. Temporozygomatic s.
- ○ 6. Nasomaxillary s.
- ○ 7. Zygomaticomaxillary s.
- 8. Infraorbital f.

- 9. Mental f.
- ○ 10. Sagittal s.
- ○ 11. Coronal s.
- 12. Supraorbital f.
- ○ 13. Frontomaxillary s.
- ○ 14. Frontonasal s.
- ○ 15. Internasal s.
- 16. Teeth

Key of abbreviations
s. Suture
f. Foramen

The SKELETAL System

Axial skeleton

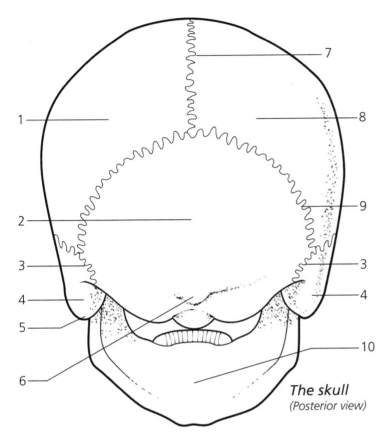

The skull
(Posterior view)

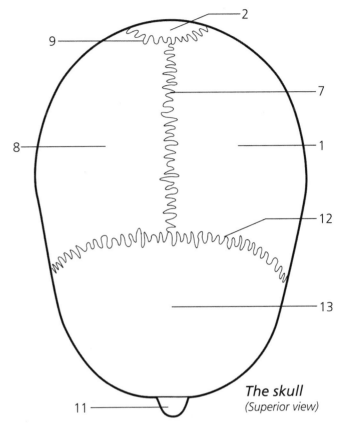

The skull
(Superior view)

○ 1. Left parietal bone
○ 2. Occipital bone
○ 3. Squamous suture
○ 4. Temporal bone
– 5. Mastoid process

– 6. External occipital process
○ 7. Sagittal suture
○ 8. Right parietal bone
○ 9. Lambdoid suture
○ 10. Mandible

○ 11. Nasal bones
○ 12. Coronal suture
○ 13. Frontal bone

Bones of the right ear
(Medial view)

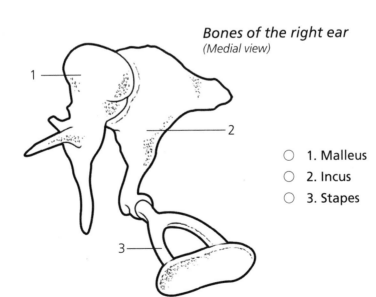

○ 1. Malleus
○ 2. Incus
○ 3. Stapes

4.7

The teeth

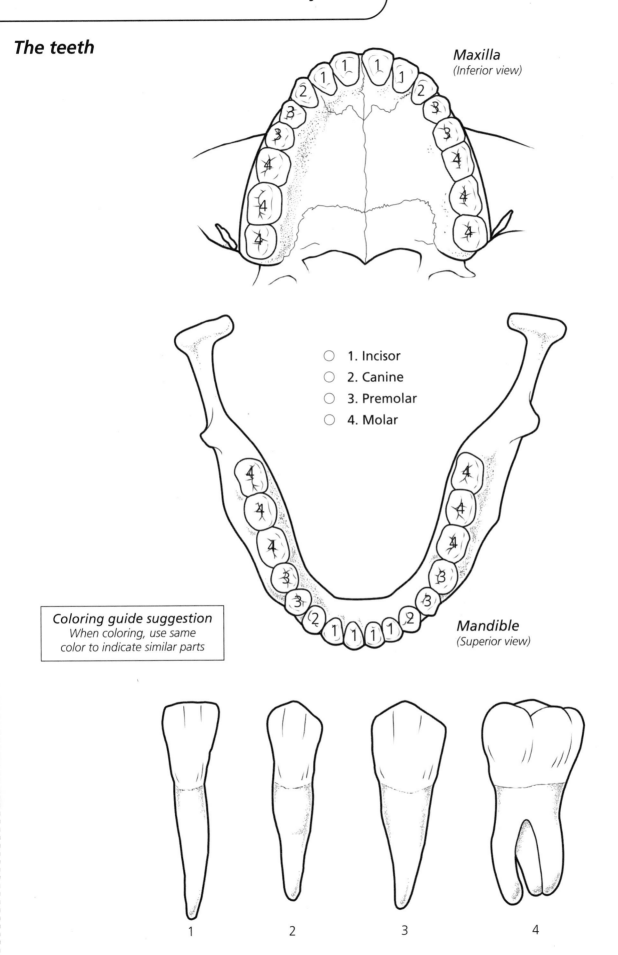

Maxilla
(Inferior view)

○ 1. Incisor
○ 2. Canine
○ 3. Premolar
○ 4. Molar

Coloring guide suggestion
*When coloring, use same
color to indicate similar parts*

Mandible
(Superior view)

1   2   3   4

The SKELETAL System

Axial skeleton

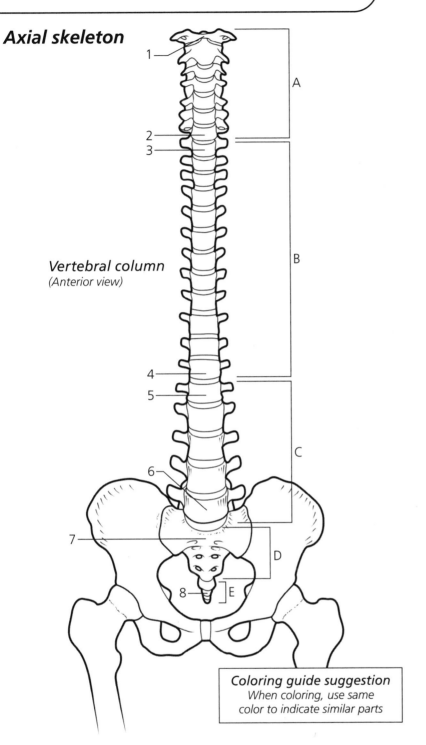

Vertebral column
(Anterior view)

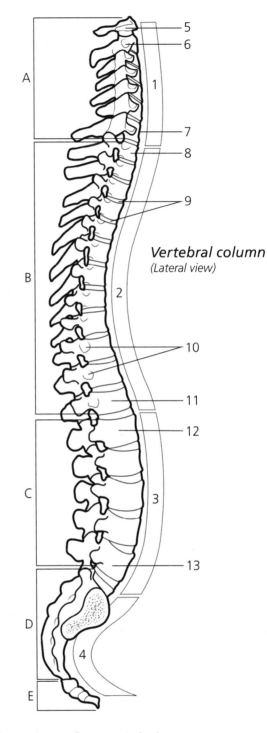

Vertebral column
(Lateral view)

Coloring guide suggestion
When coloring, use same color to indicate similar parts

A – Cervical vertebrae (C1-C7)
    ○ 1. Atlas (C1)   ○ 2. C7
B – Thoracic vertebrae (T1-T12)
    ○ 3. T1   ○ 4. T12
C – Lumbar vertebrae (L1-L5)
    ○ 5. L1   ○ 6. L5
D – Sacrum (S1-S5) *Fused*
    ○ 7. S1-S5
E – Coccyx (CO1-CO4) *Fused*
    ○ 8. CO1-CO4

A – Cervical vertebrae (C1-C7)
B – Thoracic vertebrae (T1-T12)
C – Lumbar vertebrae (L1-L5)
D – Sacrum (S1-S5)
E – Coccyx (CO1-CO4)
  ○ 1. Cervical curve
  ○ 2. Thoracic curve
  ○ 3. Lumbar curve
  ○ 4. Sacral curve
  ○ 5. Atlas (C1)

○ 6. Axis (C2)
○ 7. C7
○ 8. T1
○ 9. Intervertebral discs
○ 10. Foveae (*for rib articulation*)
○ 11. T12
○ 12. L1
○ 13. L5

4.9

Axial skeleton

Intervertebral disc

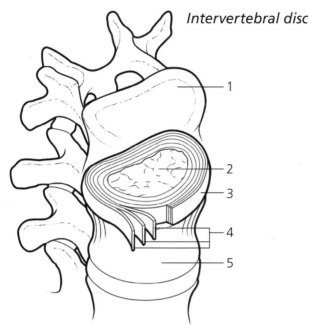

○ 1. Vertebral body (*ghosted*)
○ 2. Nucleus pulposus
○ 3. Annulus fibrosus
− 4. Concentric lamellae (*cut*)
○ 5. Vertebral body

Vertebra and spinal cord

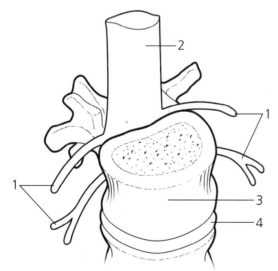

○ 1. Spinal nerves
○ 2. Spinal cord
○ 3. Vertebral body
○ 4. Intervertebral disc

Vertebral column
(*Lateral view*)

○ 1. Atlas (C1)
○ 2. Axis (C2)
○ 3. Cervical vertebrae (C1-C7)

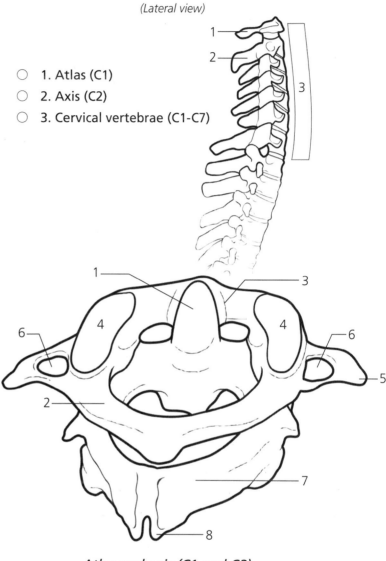

Atlas and axis (C1 and C2)
(*Posterior view*)

− 1. Dens
○ 2. Atlas
− 3. Articular facet for dens of axis
○ 4. Superior articular facet
− 5. Transverse process
− 6. Transverse foramen (*open space*)
○ 7. Axis
− 8. Spinous process

4.10

Axial skeleton

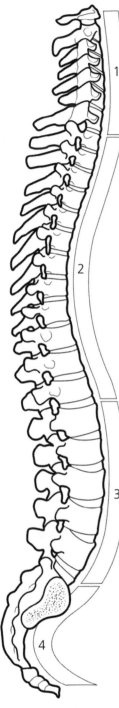

Vertebral column
(Lateral view)

○ 1. Cervical curve
○ 2. Thoracic curve
○ 3. Lumbar curve
○ 4. Sacral curve

Cervical vertebrae (C1-C7)

○ 1. Body
A – Transverse process
  – 2. Anterior tubercle
  – 3. Transverse foramen (*open space*)
  – 4. Posterior tubercle
○ 5. Superior articular facet
– 6. Pedicle
– 7. Inferior articular process
– 8. Lamina
– 9. Spinous process

Thoracic vertebrae (T1-T12)

○ 1. Body
○ 2. Superior costal facet
○ 3. Inferior costal facet (*for rib articulation*)
○ 4. Transverse costal facet
– 5. Superior articular process
○ 6. Superior articular facet
○ 7. Rib
– 8. Transverse process
– 9. Inferior articular process
– 10. Spinous process

Lumbar vertebrae (L1-L5)

○ 1. Body
– 2. Vertebral foramen (*open space for spinal cord*)
– 3. Inferior articular process
– 4. Transverse process
○ 5. Superior articular facet
– 6. Superior articular process
– 7. Spinous process

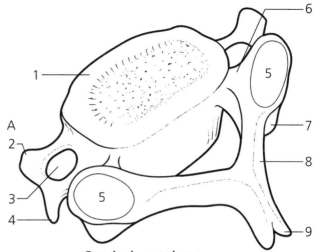

Cervical vertebrae
(Posterior view)

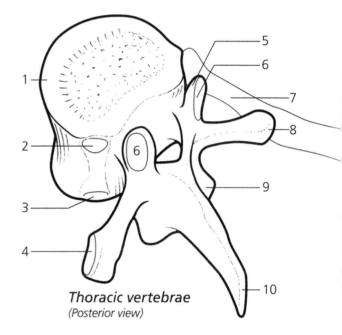

Thoracic vertebrae
(Posterior view)

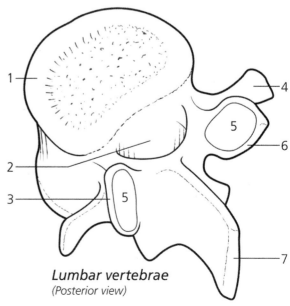

Lumbar vertebrae
(Posterior view)

4.11

Axial skeleton

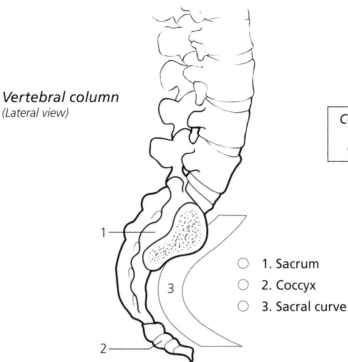

Vertebral column
(Lateral view)

> **Coloring guide suggestion**
> *When coloring, use same
> color to indicate similar parts*

○ 1. Sacrum
○ 2. Coccyx
○ 3. Sacral curve

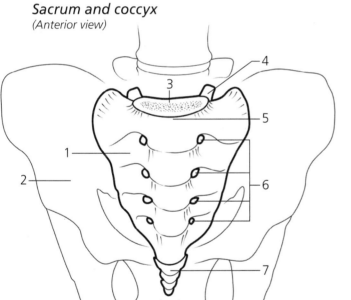

Sacrum and coccyx
(Anterior view)

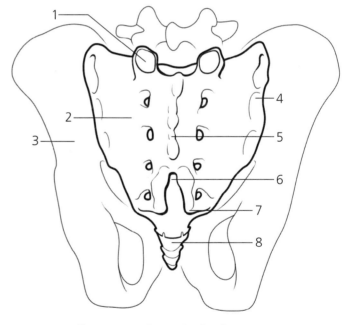

Sacrum and coccyx
(Posterior view)

○ 1. Sacrum
○ 2. Os coxae (*hip bones*)
○ 3. Base
– 4. Superior articular process
– 5. Promontory
– 6. Pelvic sacral foramina (*open space*)
○ 7. Coccyx

○ 1. Superior articular facet
○ 2. Sacrum
○ 3. Os coxae (*hip bones*)
– 4. Auricular surface (*for hip articulation*)
– 5. Median sacral crest
– 6. Sacral hiatus
– 7. Sacral cornua
○ 8. Coccyx

4.12

Appendicular skeleton

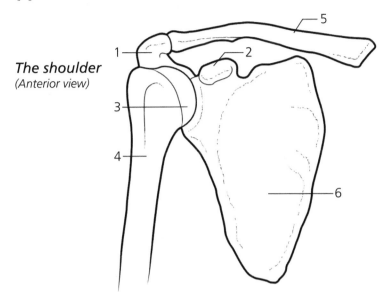

The shoulder
(Anterior view)

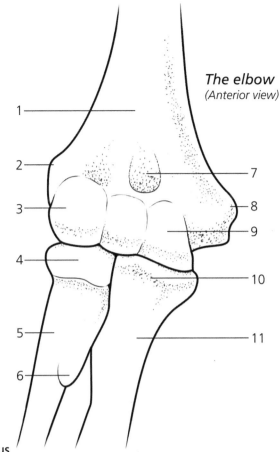

The elbow
(Anterior view)

○ 1. Acromion   ○ 4. Humerus
− 2. Coracoid process   ○ 5. Clavicle
○ 3. Head of humerus   ○ 6. Scapula

○ 1. Humerus
− 2. Lateral epicondyle
○ 3. Capitulum
○ 4. Head of radius
○ 5. Radius
− 6. Radial tuberosity
− 7. Coronoid fossa
− 8. Medial epicondyle
○ 9. Trochlea
− 10. Coronoid process
○ 11. Ulna

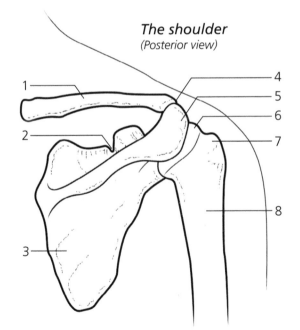

The shoulder
(Posterior view)

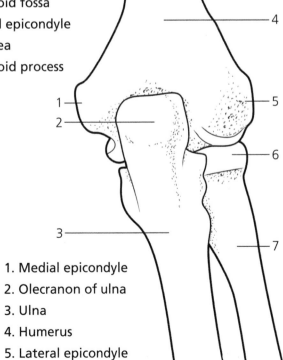

The elbow
(Posterior view)

○ 1. Clavicle   ○ 5. Acromion
− 2. Suprascapular notch   ○ 6. Head of humerus
○ 3. Scapula   − 7. Greater tubercle
− 4. Acromioclavicular joint   ○ 8. Humerus

− 1. Medial epicondyle
− 2. Olecranon of ulna
○ 3. Ulna
○ 4. Humerus
− 5. Lateral epicondyle
○ 6. Head of radius
○ 7. Radius

Coloring guide suggestion
*When coloring, use same
color to indicate similar parts*

4.13

The SKELETAL System

Appendicular skeleton

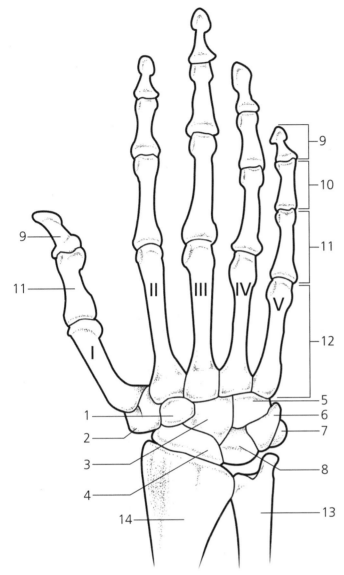

Bones of the hand and wrist
(Dorsal view)

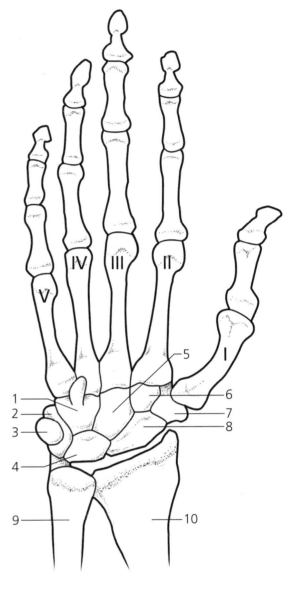

Bones of the hand and wrist
(Palmar view)

Carpal bones

- ○ 1. Trapezoid
- ○ 2. Trapezium
- ○ 3. Capitate
- ○ 4. Scaphoid
- ○ 5. Hamate
- ○ 6. Triquetrum
- ○ 7. Pisiform
- ○ 8. Lunate

Phalanges

- ○ 9. Distal phalanges
- ○ 10. Middle phalanges
- ○ 11. Proximal phalanges
- ○ 12. Metacarpals (*I through V*)
- ○ 13. Ulna
- ○ 14. Radius

Carpal bones

- ○ 1. Hamate
- ○ 2. Triquetrum
- ○ 3. Pisiform
- ○ 4. Lunate
- ○ 5. Capitate
- ○ 6. Trapezoid
- ○ 7. Trapezium
- ○ 8. Scaphoid
- ○ 9. Ulna
- ○ 10. Radius

4.14

Appendicular skeleton

The pelvic girdle
(Anterior view)

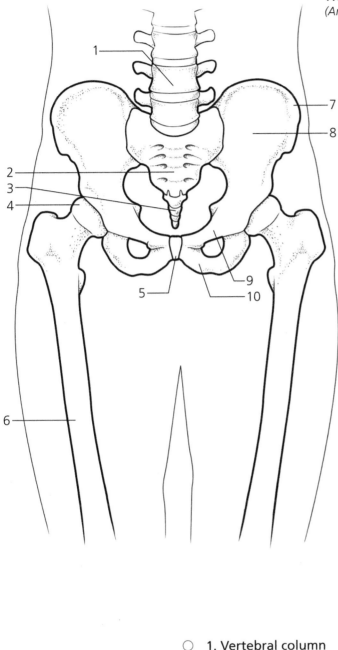

○ 1. Vertebral column
○ 2. Sacrum
○ 3. Coccyx
○ 4. Head of femur
○ 5. Pubic symphysis
○ 6. Femur
○ 7. Os coxae
   − 8. Ilium
   − 9. Pubis
   − 10. Ischium

The pelvic girdle
(Posterior view)

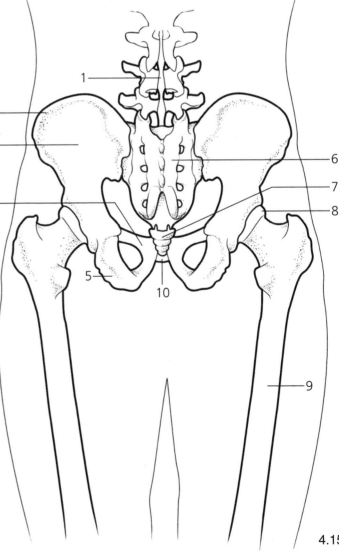

○ 1. Vertebral column
○ 2. Os coxae
   − 3. Ilium
   − 4. Pubis
   − 5. Ischium
○ 6. Sacrum
○ 7. Coccyx
○ 8. Head of femur
○ 9. Femur
○ 10. Pubic symphysis

Appendicular skeleton

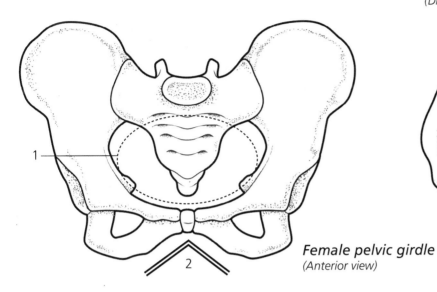

Female pelvic girdle
(Anterior view)

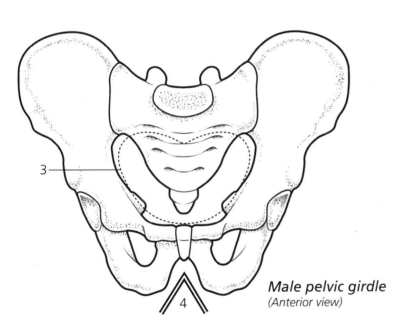

Male pelvic girdle
(Anterior view)

Femur ball and socket
(Dislocated lateral view)

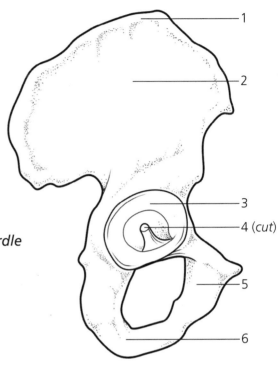

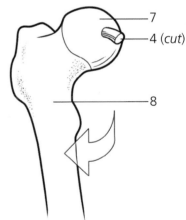

○ 1. Pelvic inlet round or oval
○ 2. Pubic arch obtuse (*greater than 90°*)
○ 3. Pelvic inlet heart-shaped
○ 4. Pubic arch acute (*less than 90°*)

○ 1. Os coxae
– 2. Ilium
○ 3. Articular lunate surface of acetabulum
○ 4. Ligament (*cut*)
– 5. Pubis
– 6. Ischium
○ 7. Head of femur
○ 8. Femur

Appendicular skeleton

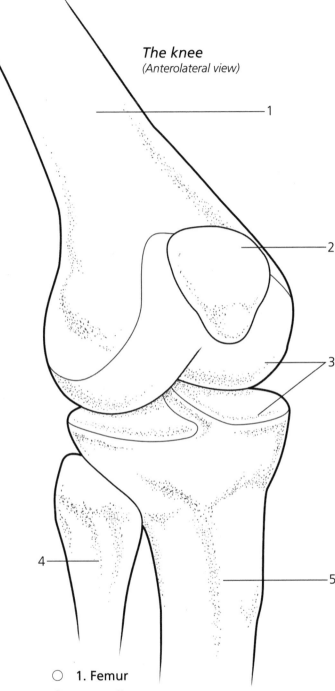

The knee
(Anterolateral view)

1

2*

3

4

5

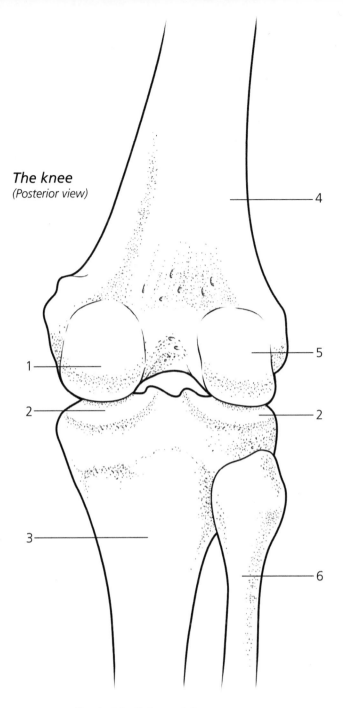

The knee
(Posterior view)

4

1

2

5

3

2

6

○ 1. Femur
○ 2. Patella*
○ 3. Articular cartilage
○ 4. Fibula
○ 5. Tibia

○ 1. Medial condyle
– 2. Articular surface
○ 3. Tibia
○ 4. Femur
○ 5. Lateral condyle
○ 6. Fibula

*Sesamoid bone
Is a bone that forms in a tendon over a joint. The patellae (kneecaps) are large sesamoid bones that all people have. Most people have extra, much smaller sesamoid bones near other joints, often in the hands and feet.

Coloring guide suggestion
When coloring, use same color to indicate similar parts

4.17

The SKELETAL System

Appendicular skeleton

- ○ 1. Tibia
- ○ 2. Fibula
- − 3. Medial malleolus
- − 4. Lateral malleolus
- ○ 5. Talus

Tarsal bones

- ○ 6. Lateral cuneiform
- ○ 7. Navicular
- ○ 8. Intermediate cuneiform
- ○ 9. Medial cuneiform
- ○ 10. Calcaneus
- ○ 11. Metatarsal bones (*I through V*)

Phalanges

- ○ 12. Proximal phalanges
- ○ 13. Middle phalanges
- ○ 14. Distal phalanges
- ○ 15. Sesamoid bones*
- ○ 16. Cuboid

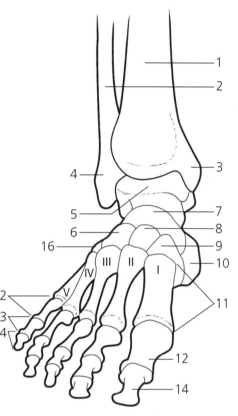

Bones of the right foot
(Anterior view)

Bones of the right foot
(Plantar view)

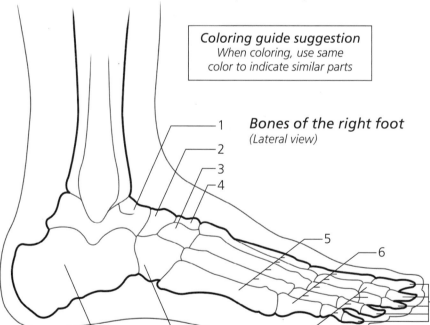

Coloring guide suggestion
When coloring, use same color to indicate similar parts

Bones of the right foot
(Lateral view)

*Sesamoid bone
Is a bone that forms in a tendon over a joint. Most people have extra, much smaller sesamoid bones near other joints, often in the hands and feet.

- ○ 1. Talus
- ○ 2. Navicular
- ○ 3. Lateral cuneiform
- ○ 4. Intermediate cuneiform
- ○ 5. Metatarsals
- ○ 6. Proximal phalanges
- ○ 7. Middle phalanges
- ○ 8. Distal phalanges
- ○ 9. Calcaneus
- ○ 10. Cuboid

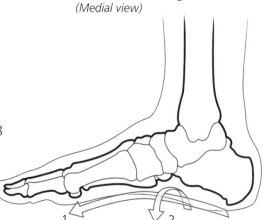

Arches of the right foot
(Medial view)

- ○ 1. Longitudinal arch
- ○ 2. Transverse arch

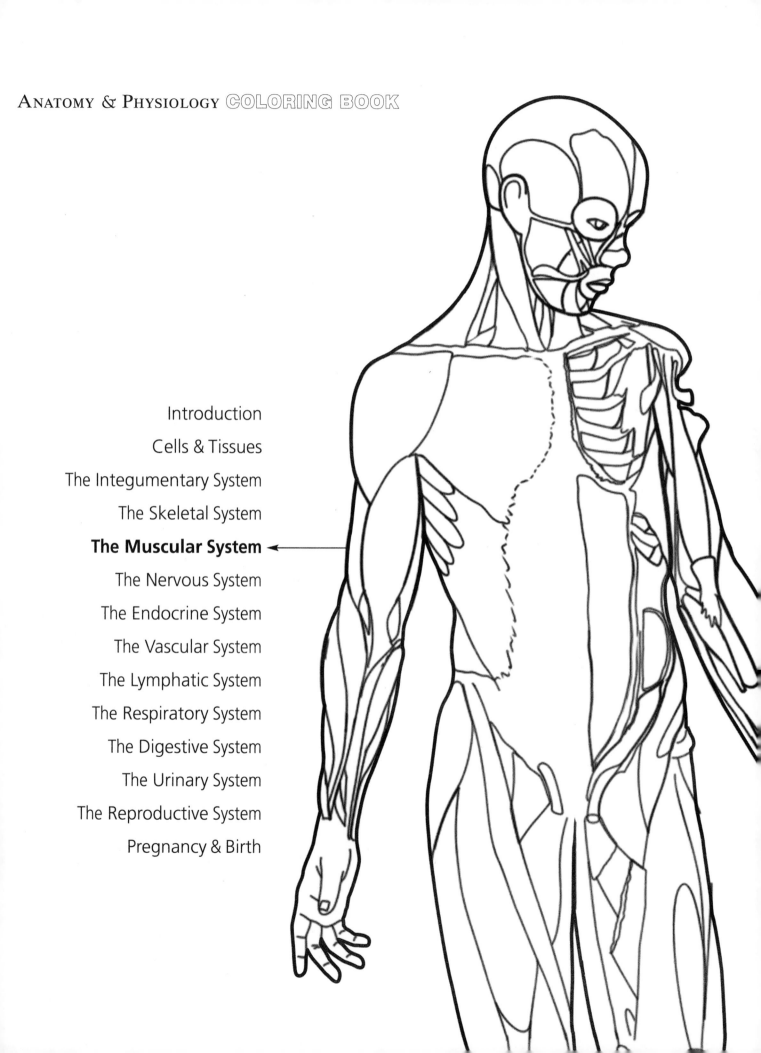

ANATOMY & PHYSIOLOGY COLORING BOOK

The MUSCULAR System

System overview

The muscular system interacts with the skeletal system to allow us to produce a wide variety of motions, including dancing, sitting and breathing. Skeletal muscle provides the power that enables us to move under conscious control. Additionally, skeletal muscle provides the force needed to move venous blood back to the heart.

Skeletal muscle structure

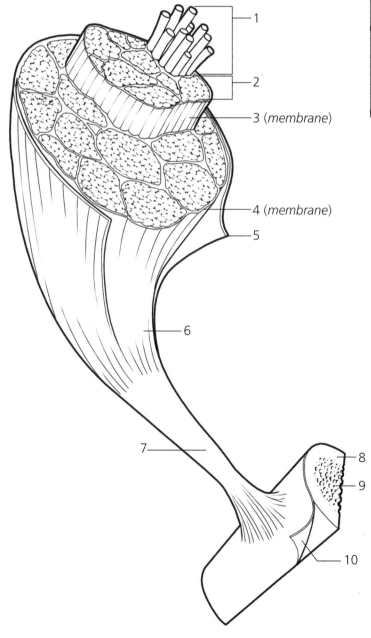

Types of muscle

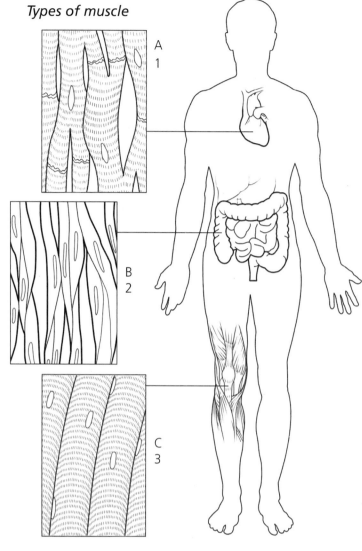

A – Cardiac
  ○ 1. Heart

B – Smooth
  ○ 2. Digestive organs

C – Skeletal
  ○ 3. Joints (*all voluntary muscle*)

○ 1. Muscle fibers
○ 2. Muscle fascicle
– 3. Perimysium (*membrane*)
– 4. Epimysium (*membrane*)
○ 5. Fascia

○ 6. Skeletal muscle
○ 7. Tendon
○ 8. Compact bone
○ 9. Spongy bone
○ 10. Periosteum (*covering the bone*)

5.1

Skeletal muscle structure

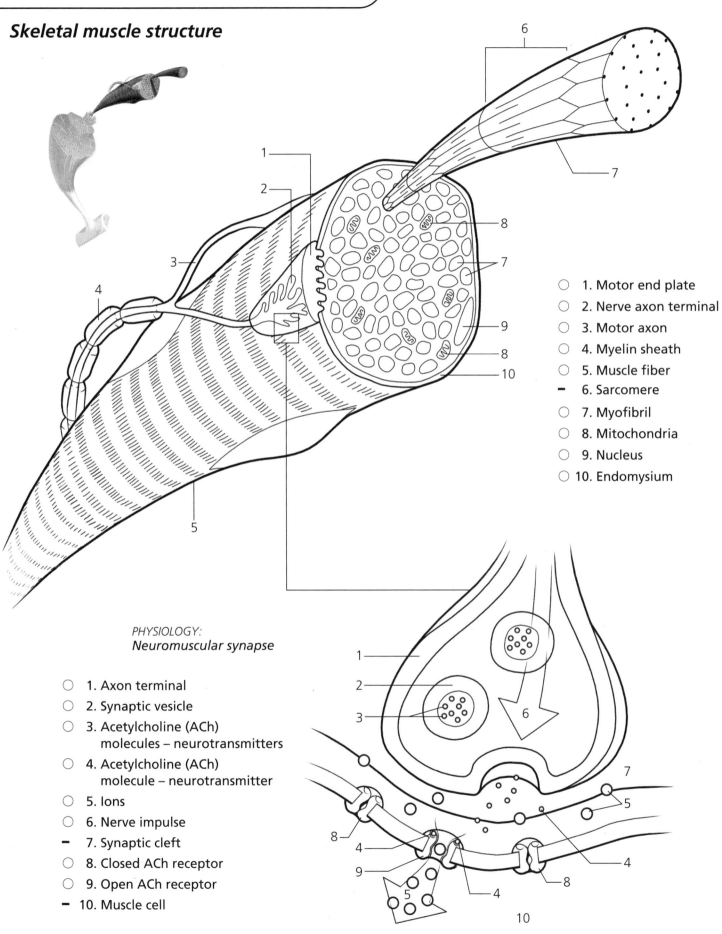

○ 1. Motor end plate
○ 2. Nerve axon terminal
○ 3. Motor axon
○ 4. Myelin sheath
○ 5. Muscle fiber
– 6. Sarcomere
○ 7. Myofibril
○ 8. Mitochondria
○ 9. Nucleus
○ 10. Endomysium

PHYSIOLOGY:
Neuromuscular synapse

○ 1. Axon terminal
○ 2. Synaptic vesicle
○ 3. Acetylcholine (ACh)
   molecules – neurotransmitters
○ 4. Acetylcholine (ACh)
   molecule – neurotransmitter
○ 5. Ions
○ 6. Nerve impulse
– 7. Synaptic cleft
○ 8. Closed ACh receptor
○ 9. Open ACh receptor
– 10. Muscle cell

The MUSCULAR System

Surface anatomy: Anterior

Male
(Anterior view)

○ 1. Auris (*ear*)
○ 2. Bucca (*cheek*)
○ 3. Cervical (*neck*)
○ 4. Axilla (*armpit*)
○ 5. Brachium (arm)
○ 6. Antecubitis (*front of elbow*)
○ 7. Antebrachium (*forearm*)
○ 8. Inguen (*groin*)
○ 9. Pubis
○ 10. Manus (*hand*)
○ 11. Femur (*thigh*)
○ 12. Patella (*kneecap*)
○ 13. Crus (*leg*)
○ 14. Tarsus (*ankle*)
○ 15. Digits (*toes*)
○ 16. Hallux (*big toe*)

○ 17. Frons (*forehead*)
○ 18. Oculus (*eye*)
○ 19. Nasus (*nose*)
○ 20. Oris (*mouth*)
○ 21. Mentis (*chin*)
○ 22. Cranium (*skull*)
○ 23. Facies (*face*)
○ 24. Cephalon (*head*)
○ 25. Thoracis (*chest*)
○ 26. Mamma (*breast*)
○ 27. Abdomen
○ 28. Umbilicus (*navel*)
○ 29. Pelvis
○ 30. Trunk
○ 31. Carpus (*wrist*)
○ 32. Pollex (*thumb*)
○ 33. Palma (*palm*)
○ 34. Digits (*fingers*)
○ 35. Pes (*foot*)

The MUSCULAR System

Surface anatomy: Posterior

○ 1. Deltoid (*shoulder*)
○ 2. Dorsum (*back*)
○ 3. Olecranon (*back of elbow*)
○ 4. Lumbus (*loin*)
○ 5. Gluteus (*buttock*)
○ 6. Popliteus (*back of knee*)
○ 7. Sura (*calf*)
○ 8. Plantar (*sole of foot*)
○ 9. Calcaneus (*heel of foot*)
○ 10. Cephalon (*head*)
○ 11. Cervicis (*neck*)
○ 12. Upper limb
○ 13. Lower limb

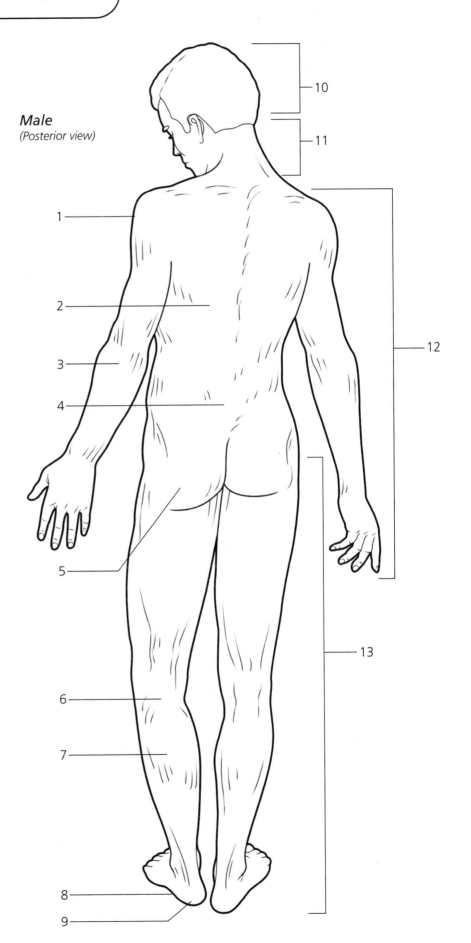

Male
(Posterior view)

The MUSCULAR System

Key of abbreviations
m. Muscle

Anterior: Muscle anatomy

Head and neck
(Anterolateral view – superficial)

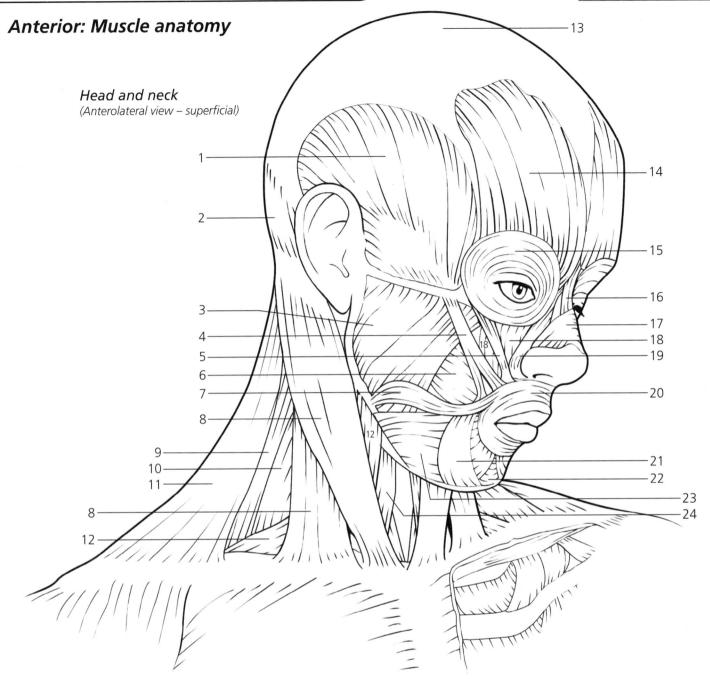

○ 1. Temporalis m.

○ 2. Occipitalis m. (*part of epicranius*)

○ 3. Masseter m.

○ 4. Zygomaticus major m.

○ 5. Zygomaticus minor m.

○ 6. Buccinator m.

○ 7. Risorius m.

○ 8. Sternocleidomastoid m.

○ 9. Middle scalene m.

○ 10. Anterior scalene m.

○ 11. Trapezius m.

○ 12. Omohyoid m.

– 13. Aponeurosis of epicranius (*Galea aponeurotica*)

○ 14. Frontalis m. (*part of epicranius*)

○ 15. Orbicularis oculi m.

○ 16. Procerus m.

○ 17. Nasalis m.

○ 18. Levator labii superioris m.

○ 19. Levator labii superioris alaeque nasi m.

○ 20. Orbicularis oris m.

○ 21. Depressor anguli oris m.

○ 22. Mentalis m.

○ 23. Platysma m.

○ 24. Sternohyoid m.

The MUSCULAR System

Anterior: Muscle anatomy

Chest & abdomen
(Anterior view – superficial)

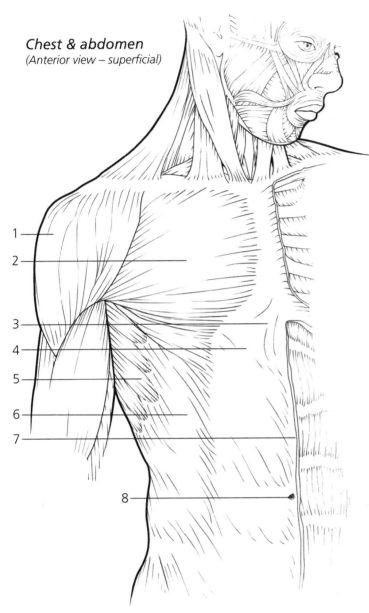

Chest & abdomen
(Anterior view – deep)

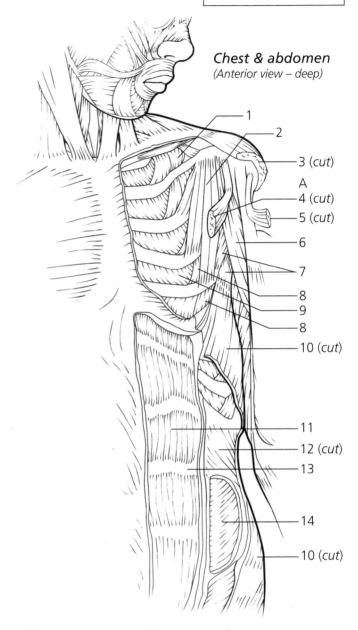

○ 1. Deltoid m.
○ 2. Pectoralis major m.
– 3. Costoxiphoid ll.
○ 4. Rectus sheath (*aponeurosis*)
○ 5. Serratus anterior m.
○ 6. External abdominal oblique m.
– 7. Linea alba
– 8. Umbilicus (*navel*)

○ 1. Serratus anterior m., superior part
○ 2. Pectoralis minor m.
○ 3. Deltoid m. (*cut*)
A – Biceps m.: (*cut*)
   ○ 4. Short head   ○ 5. Long head
○ 6. Coracobrachialis m.
○ 7. Serratus anterior m.
○ 8. External intercostal m.
○ 9. Internal intercostal m.
○ 10. External abdominal oblique m. (*cut*)
○ 11. Rectus abdominis m.
○ 12. Internal abdominal oblique m. (*cut*)
– 13. Tendinous inscriptions
○ 14. Transversus abdominis m.

Anterior: Muscle anatomy

Abdominal wall
(Anterior view – superficial)

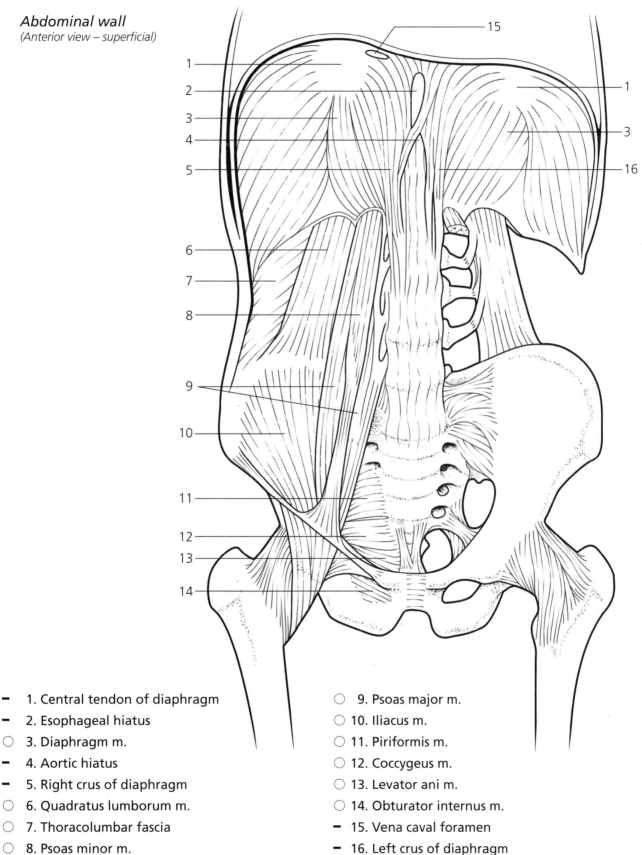

1. Central tendon of diaphragm
2. Esophageal hiatus
3. Diaphragm m.
4. Aortic hiatus
5. Right crus of diaphragm
6. Quadratus lumborum m.
7. Thoracolumbar fascia
8. Psoas minor m.

9. Psoas major m.
10. Iliacus m.
11. Piriformis m.
12. Coccygeus m.
13. Levator ani m.
14. Obturator internus m.
15. Vena caval foramen
16. Left crus of diaphragm

Anterior: Muscle anatomy

Arm
(Anterior view – superficial)

Key of abbreviations
m. Muscle

○ 1. Deltoid m.

A – Biceps m.:

    ○ 2. Long head

    ○ 3. Short head

B – Triceps m.:

    ○ 4. Long head

    ○ 5. Medial head

○ 6. Brachialis m.

○ 7. Brachioradialis m.

○ 8. Extensor carpi radialis longus m.

○ 9. Flexor digitorum superficialis m.

○ 10. Abductor pollicis longus m.

○ 11. Flexor pollicis longus m.

○ 12. Pronator teres m.

○ 13. Palmaris longus m.

○ 14. Flexor carpi radialis m.

○ 15. Flexor carpi ulnaris m.

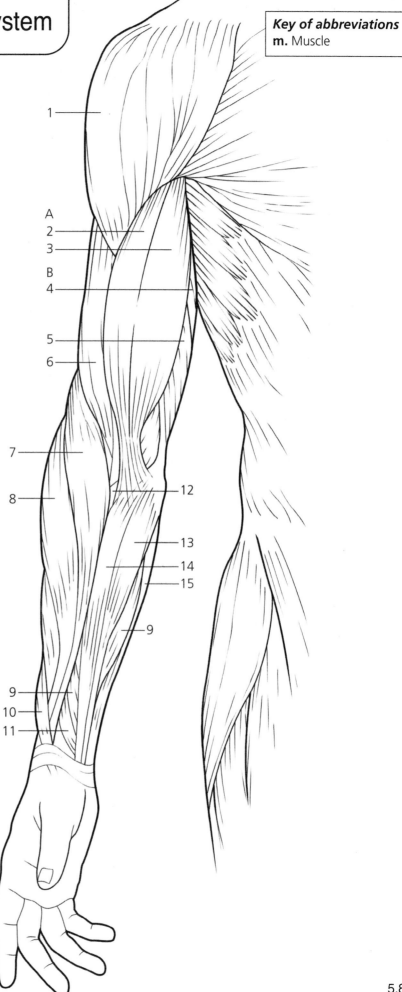

The MUSCULAR System

Key of abbreviations
m. Muscle
tt. Tendons

Anterior: Muscle anatomy

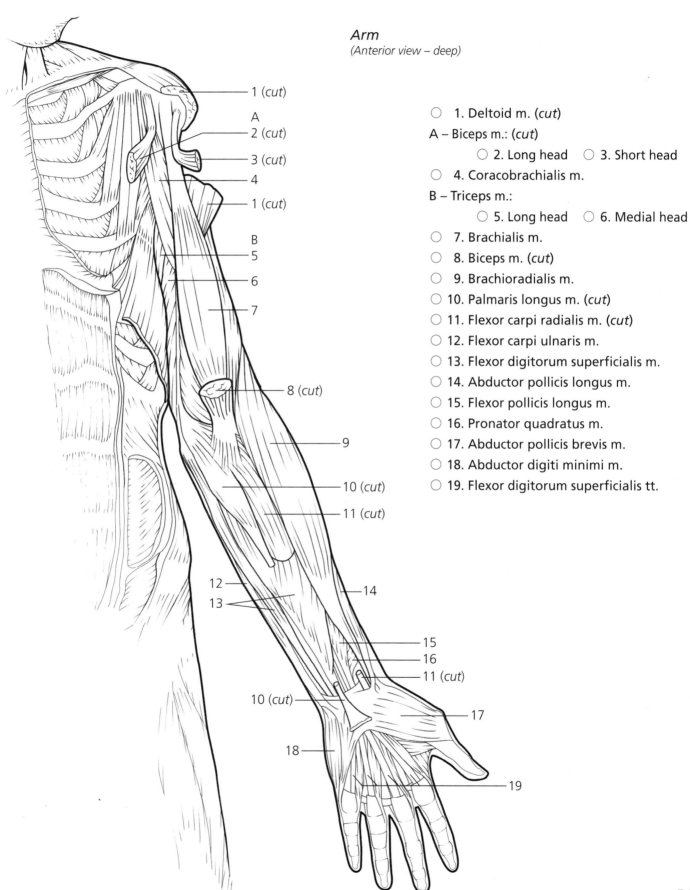

Arm
(Anterior view – deep)

○ 1. Deltoid m. *(cut)*
A – Biceps m.: *(cut)*
    ○ 2. Long head   ○ 3. Short head
○ 4. Coracobrachialis m.
B – Triceps m.:
    ○ 5. Long head   ○ 6. Medial head
○ 7. Brachialis m.
○ 8. Biceps m. *(cut)*
○ 9. Brachioradialis m.
○ 10. Palmaris longus m. *(cut)*
○ 11. Flexor carpi radialis m. *(cut)*
○ 12. Flexor carpi ulnaris m.
○ 13. Flexor digitorum superficialis m.
○ 14. Abductor pollicis longus m.
○ 15. Flexor pollicis longus m.
○ 16. Pronator quadratus m.
○ 17. Abductor pollicis brevis m.
○ 18. Abductor digiti minimi m.
○ 19. Flexor digitorum superficialis tt.

The MUSCULAR System

Key of abbreviations
m. Muscle   **t.** Tendon
l. Ligament

Anterior: Muscle anatomy

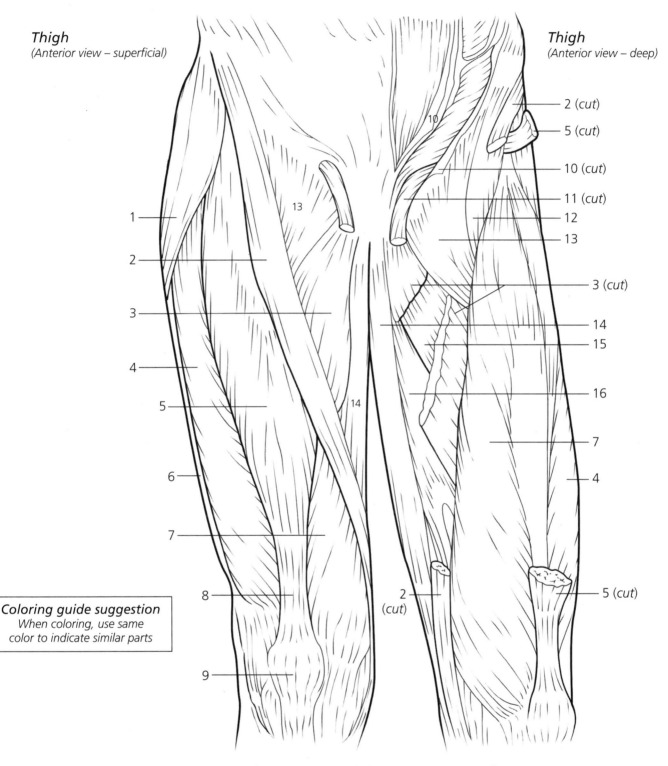

Thigh
(Anterior view – superficial)

Thigh
(Anterior view – deep)

2 (*cut*)
5 (*cut*)
10 (*cut*)
11 (*cut*)
12
13
3 (*cut*)
14
15
16
7
4
5 (*cut*)
2 (*cut*)

13
10
14

1
2
3
4
5
6
7
8
9

Coloring guide suggestion
When coloring, use same color to indicate similar parts

○ 1. Tensor fasciae latae m.
○ 2. Sartorius m.
○ 3. Adductor longus m.
○ 4. Vastus lateralis m.
○ 5. Rectus femoris m.
– 6. Iliotibial tract

○ 7. Vastus medialis m.
– 8. Rectus femoris t. (*quadriceps t.*)
– 9. Patellar l.
○ 10. Inguinal l. (*cut*)
○ 11. Cremaster m. (*cut*)
○ 12. Iliopsoas m.

○ 13. Pectineus m.
○ 14. Gracilis m.
○ 15. Adductor brevis m.
○ 16. Adductor magnus m.

5.10

Key of abbreviations
m. Muscle **t.** Tendon
l. Ligament

Anterior: Muscle anatomy

Lower leg and foot
(Anterior view – superficial)

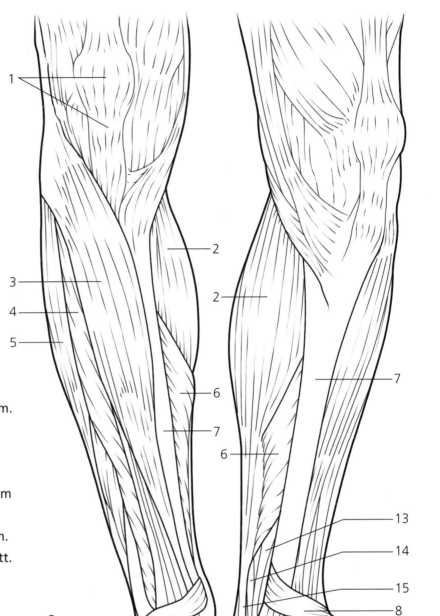

— 1. Patellar l.
○ 2. Gastrocnemius m.
○ 3. Tibialis anterior m.
○ 4. Extensor digitorum longus m.
○ 5. Peroneus longus m.
○ 6. Soleus m.
— 7. Tibia
○ 8. Inferior extensor retinaculum
○ 9. Extensor hallucis brevis m.
○ 10. Extensor digitorum brevis m.
○ 11. Extensor digitorum longus tt.
○ 12. Extensor hallucis longus m.
○ 13. Flexor digitorum longus m.
○ 14. Flexor hallucis longus m.
○ 15. Calcaneal t. (*Achilles t.*)
○ 16. Flexor retinaculum l.
○ 17. Tibialis anterior t.
○ 18. Abductor hallucis m.

The MUSCULAR System

Anterior: Muscle anatomy

Foot and ankle
(Anterior view - superficial)

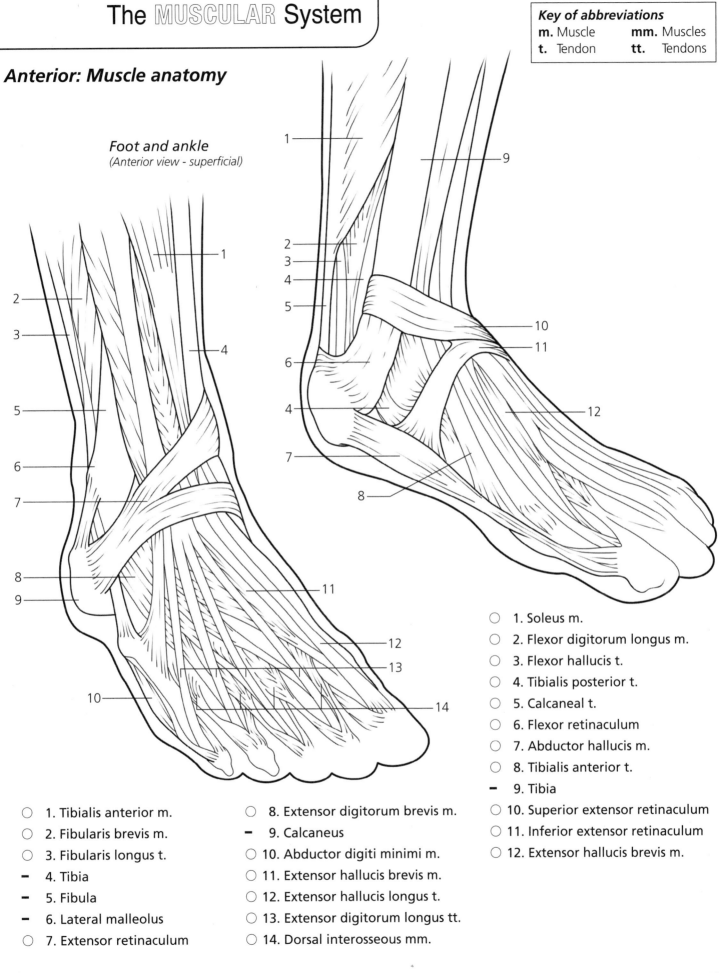

○ 1. Tibialis anterior m.
○ 2. Fibularis brevis m.
○ 3. Fibularis longus t.
–   4. Tibia
–   5. Fibula
–   6. Lateral malleolus
○ 7. Extensor retinaculum

○ 8. Extensor digitorum brevis m.
–   9. Calcaneus
○ 10. Abductor digiti minimi m.
○ 11. Extensor hallucis brevis m.
○ 12. Extensor hallucis longus t.
○ 13. Extensor digitorum longus tt.
○ 14. Dorsal interosseous mm.

○ 1. Soleus m.
○ 2. Flexor digitorum longus m.
○ 3. Flexor hallucis t.
○ 4. Tibialis posterior t.
○ 5. Calcaneal t.
○ 6. Flexor retinaculum
○ 7. Abductor hallucis m.
○ 8. Tibialis anterior t.
–   9. Tibia
○ 10. Superior extensor retinaculum
○ 11. Inferior extensor retinaculum
○ 12. Extensor hallucis brevis m.

5.12

The MUSCULAR System

Posterior: Muscle anatomy

Head and neck
(Posterior view – superficial)

9
10
11
1
12
2
13
3
14
4
15
5
16
6
17
7
18
8
19

○ 1. Frontalis m.
○ 2. Orbicularis oculi m.
○ 3. Zygomaticus major m.
○ 4. Masseter m.
○ 5. Orbicularis oris m.
○ 6. Risorius m.
○ 7. Depressor anguli oris m.
○ 8. Trapezius m.
○ 9. Galea aponeurotica (*epicraneal aponeurosis*)
○ 10. Temporalis m.

○ 11. Occipitalis m.
○ 12. Posterior auricular m.
○ 13. Splenius m.
○ 14. Sternocleidomastoid m.
○ 15. Longissimus capitis m.
○ 16. Splenius capitis m.
○ 17. Splenius cervicis m.
○ 18. Levator scapulae m.
○ 19. Rhomboid minor m.

The MUSCULAR System

Key of abbreviations
m. Muscle

Posterior: Muscle anatomy

Back and upper arm
(Posterior view – superficial)

○ 1. Trapezius m.
○ 2. Deltoid m.
○ 3. Infraspinatus m.
○ 4. Teres minor m.
○ 5. Teres major m.
A – Triceps m.:
      ○ 6. Lateral head
      ○ 7. Long head
○ 8. Latissimus dorsi m.
○ 9. Brachialis m.
○ 10. Brachioradialis m.

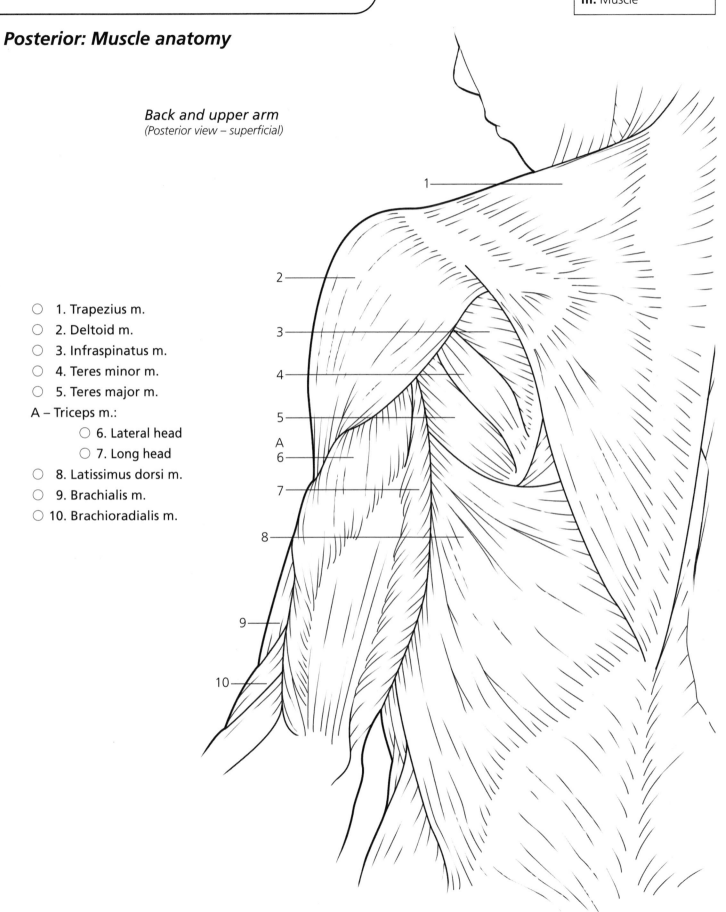

Key of abbreviations
m. Muscle

Posterior: Muscle anatomy

Back
(Posterior view – deep)

○   1. Levator scapulae m.
○   2. Rhomboid minor m.
○   3. Rhomboid major m.
○   4. Supraspinatus m.
○   5. Infraspinatus m.
○   6. Teres minor m.
○   7. Spinalis thoracis m.
○   8. Longissimus thoracis m.
○   9. Teres major m.
○ 10. Iliocostalis thoracis m.
○ 11. Serratus anterior m.
○ 12. Serratus posterior inferior m.
○ 13. Thoracolumbar fascia (*cut*)
○ 14. External oblique m.

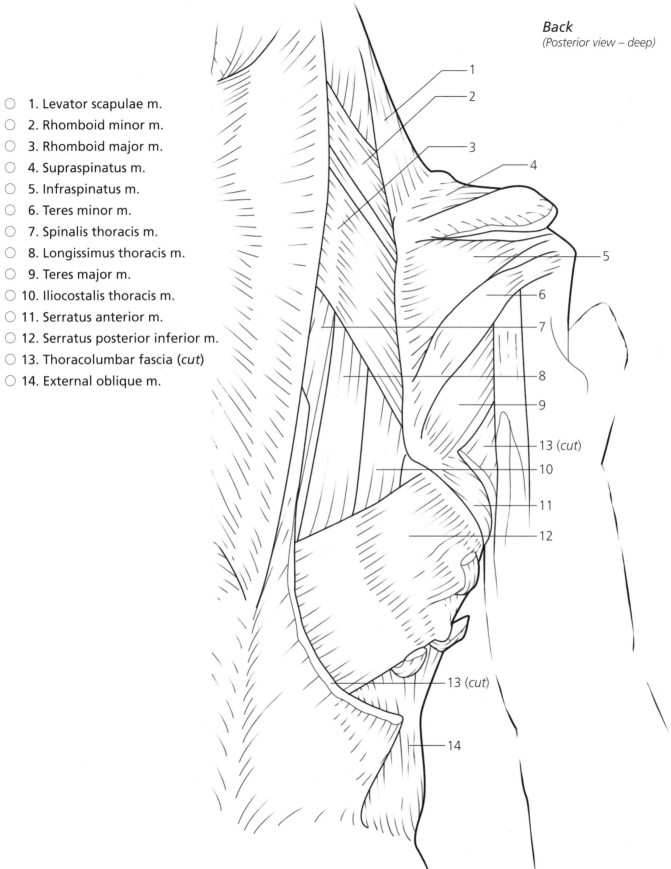

The MUSCULAR System

Key of abbreviations
m. Muscle
mm. Muscles

Posterior: Muscle anatomy

Back
(Posterior view – deep)

1. Semispinalis capitis m.
2. Longissimus capitis m.
3. Splenius cervicis m.
4. C7 vertebra
5. Semispinalis thoracis m.
6. Intertransversarii thoracis mm.
7. Levatores costarum breves mm.
8. Levatores costarum longi mm.
9. Intertransversarii lumborum mm.
10. Multifidus mm.
11. Splenius capitis m.
12. Levator scapulae m. (*cut*)
13. Longissimus cervicis m.
14. Spinalis thoracis m.
15. Longissimus thoracis m.
16. Iliocostalis thoracis m.
17. Iliocostalis lumborum m.
18. L1 vertebra
19. Erector spinae m.

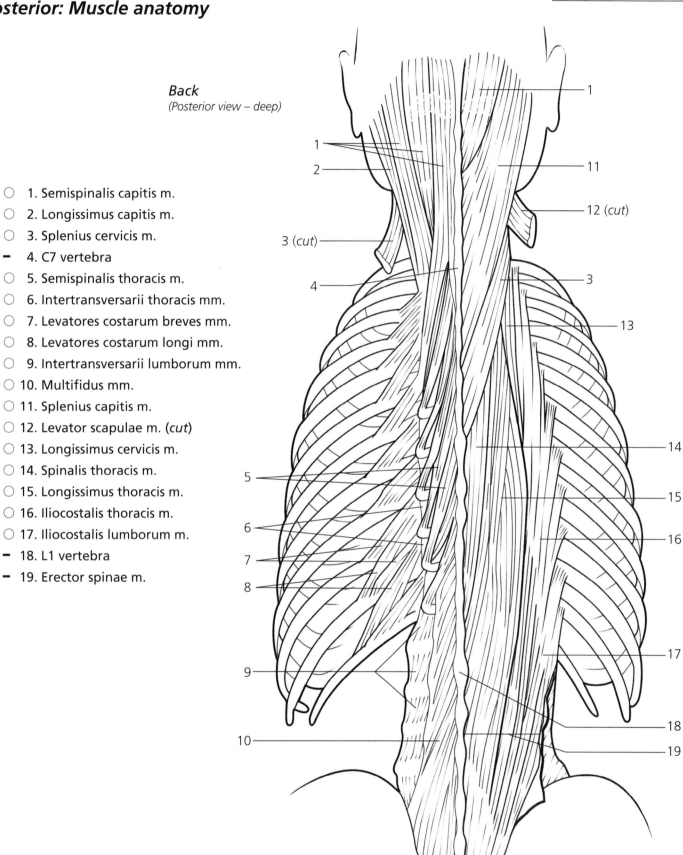

5.16

The MUSCULAR System

Posterior: Muscle anatomy

Upper arm and forearm
(Posterior view – deep)

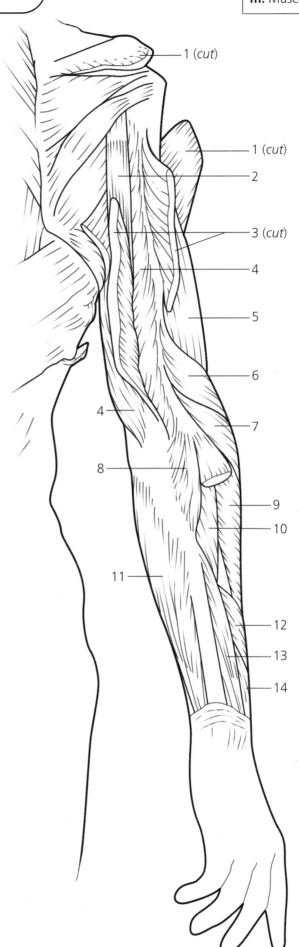

1. Deltoid m. (*cut*)
2. Triceps m., long head
3. Triceps m., lateral head (*cut*)
4. Triceps m., medial head
5. Brachialis m.
6. Brachioradialis m.
7. Extensor carpi radialis longus m.
8. Anconeus m.
9. Extensor carpi radialis brevis m.
10. Supinator m.
11. Flexor carpi ulnaris m.
12. Abductor pollicis longus m.
13. Extensor pollicis longus m.
14. Extensor pollicis brevis m.

5.17

The MUSCULAR System

Key of abbreviations
m. Muscle
mm. Muscles

Posterior: Muscle anatomy

Upper arm and forearm
(Posterior view – superficial)

○ 1. Deltoid m.

A – Triceps m.:

    ○ 2. Lateral head

    ○ 3. Long head

○ 4. Brachialis m.

○ 5. Brachioradialis m.

− 6. Olecranon process

○ 7. Extensor carpi radialis longus m.

○ 8. Anconeus m.

○ 9. Extensor digitorum m.

○ 10. Flexor carpi ulnaris m.

○ 11. Extensor carpi ulnaris m.

○ 12. Extensor carpi radialis brevis m.

○ 13. Abductor pollicis longus m.

○ 14. Extensor pollicis brevis m.

○ 15. Extensor pollicis brevis t.

○ 16. Extensor pollicis longus t.

○ 17. Dorsal interosseous mm.

○ 18. Extensor retinaculum

○ 19. Extensor digiti minimi t.

○ 20. Extensor digitorum tt.

5.18

The MUSCULAR System

Posterior: Muscle anatomy

Hips and upper legs
(Posterior view – superficial)

Hips and upper legs
(Posterior view – deep)

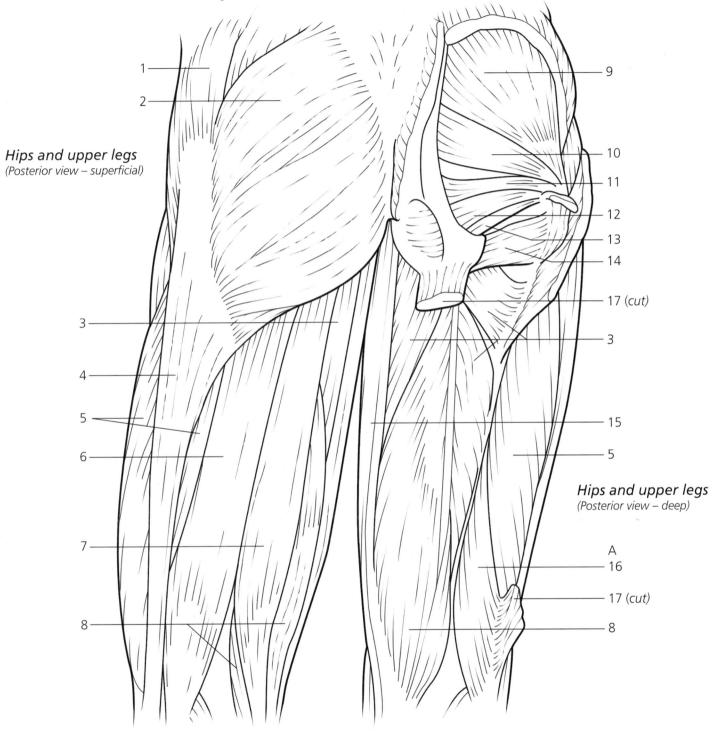

○ 1. Gluteus medius m.
○ 2. Gluteus maximus m.
○ 3. Adductor magnus m.
○ 4. Iliotibial tract
○ 5. Vastus lateralis m.
○ 6. Biceps femoris m.

○ 7. Semitendinosus m.
○ 8. Semimembranosus m.
○ 9. Gluteus minimus m.
○ 10. Piriformis m.
○ 11. Superior gemellus m.
○ 12. Obturator internus m.

○ 13. Inferior gemellus m.
○ 14. Quadratus femoris m.
○ 15. Gracilis m.
A – Biceps femoris m.:
   ○ 16. Short head
   ○ 17. long head *(cut)*

Posterior: Muscle anatomy

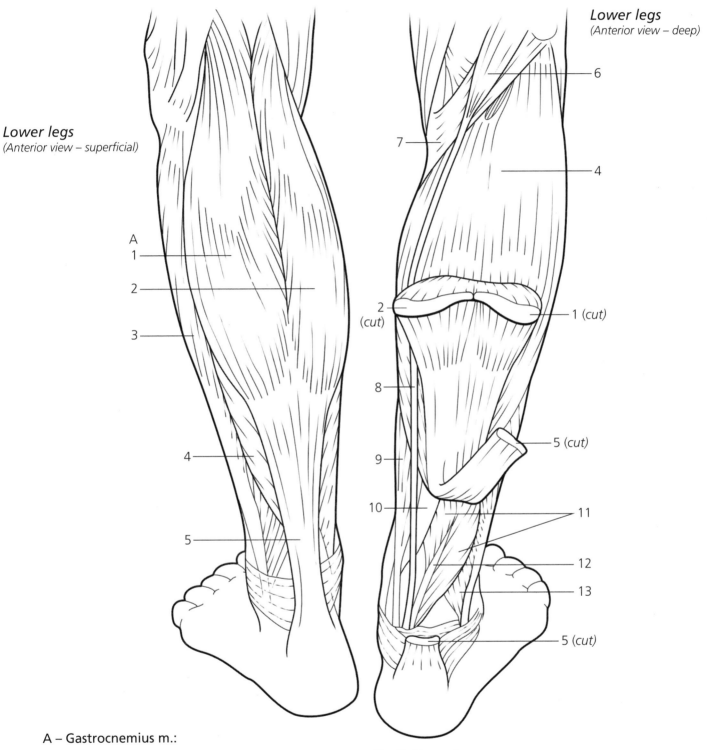

Lower legs
(Anterior view – superficial)

Lower legs
(Anterior view – deep)

A – Gastrocnemius m.:

○ 1. Lateral head

○ 2. Medial head

○ 3. Peroneus longus m. (*fibularis longus m.*)

○ 4. Soleus m.

○ 5. Calcaneal t.

○ 6. Plantaris m.

○ 7. Popliteus m.

○ 8. Plantaris t.

○ 9. Flexor digitorum longus m.

○ 10. Tibialis posterior m.

○ 11. Flexor hallucis longus m.

○ 12. Flexor hallucis longus t.

○ 13. Peroneus brevis m. (*fibularis brevis m.*)

5.20

Key of abbreviations
m. Muscle   **mm.** Muscles
t. Tendon   **tt.** Tendons

Muscle anatomy: Hand & wrist

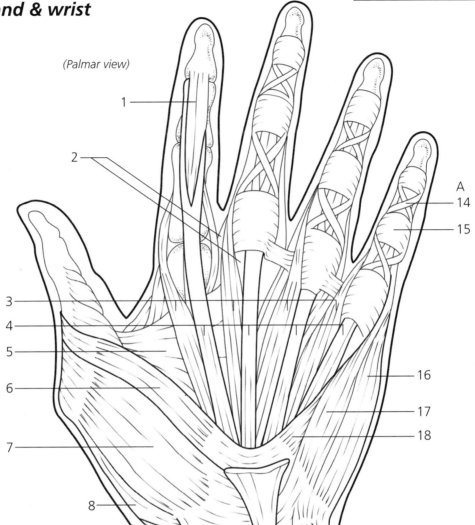

(Palmar view)

A

○ 1. Flexor digitorum profundus t.
○ 2. Palmar interosseous mm.
○ 3. Lumbrical mm.
○ 4. Flexor digitorum superficialis tt.
○ 5. Adductor pollicis m.
○ 6. Flexor pollicis brevis m.
○ 7. Abductor pollicis brevis m.
○ 8. Opponens pollicis m.
○ 9. Abductor pollicis longus t.
○ 10. Palmaris longus t.
○ 11. Flexor pollicis longus m.
○ 12. Flexor carpi radialis t.
○ 13. Brachioradialis t.
A – Fibrous digital sheath:
    ○ 14. Cruciform part
    ○ 15. Anular part

○ 16. Abductor digiti minimi m.
○ 17. Flexor digiti minimi brevis m.
○ 18. Opponens digiti minimi m.
○ 19. Flexor carpi ulnaris t.
– 20. Flexor digitorum superficialis mm. & tt.

The MUSCULAR System

Key of abbreviations
m. Muscle   **mm.** Muscles
tt. Tendons

Muscle anatomy: Hand & wrist

(Dorsal view)

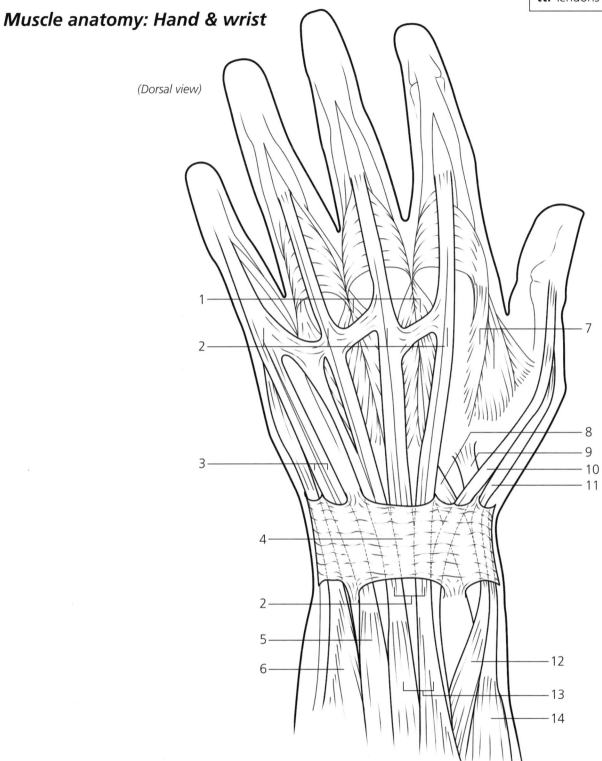

○ 1. 2nd, 3rd, 4th dorsal interosseous mm.
○ 2. Extensor digitorum tt.
○ 3. Extensor digiti minimi tt.
○ 4. Extensor retinaculum
○ 5. Extensor digiti minimi m.
○ 6. Extensor carpi ulnaris m.
○ 7. 1st dorsal interosseous m.

○ 8. Extensor carpi radialis longus t.
○ 9. Extensor carpi radialis brevis t.
○ 10. Extensor pollicis longus t.
○ 11. Extensor pollicis brevis t.
○ 12. Extensor pollicis brevis m.
○ 13. Extensor digitorum m.
○ 14. Abductor pollicis longus m.

Joint anatomy

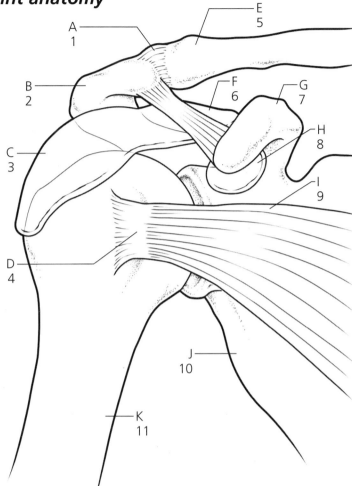

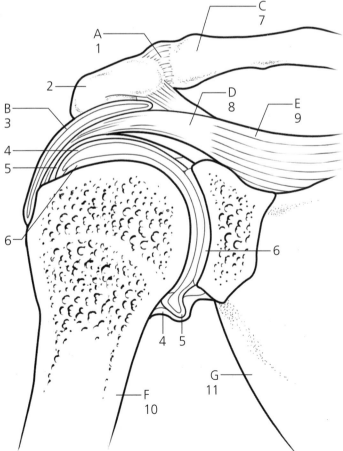

Glenohumeral joint
(Anterior view)

A – Ligament
- ○ 1. Acromioclavicular

B – Bone
- ‒ 2. Acromion of scapula

C – Bursa
- ○ 3. Subdeltoid

D – Tendon
- ○ 4. Subscapularis

E – Bone
- ‒ 5. Clavicle

F – Bursa
- ○ 6. Subacromial

G – Bone
- ‒ 7. Coracoid process of scapula

H – Bursa
- ○ 8. Subcoracoid

I – Muscle
- ○ 9. Subscapularis

J – Bone
- ‒ 10. Scapula

K – Bone
- ‒ 11. Humerus

Glenohumeral joint
(Anterior view – partial cutaway)

A – Ligament
- ○ 1. Acromioclavicular
- ‒ 2. Acromion

B – Bursa
- ○ 3. Subdeltoid
- ○ 4. Synovial membrane
- ○ 5. Joint capsule
- ○ 6. Articular cartilage

C – Bone
- ‒ 7. Clavicle

D – Tendon
- ○ 8. Supraspinatus

E – Muscle
- ○ 9. Supraspinatus

F – Bone
- ‒ 10. Humerus

G – Bone
- ‒ 11. Scapula

5.23

The MUSCULAR System

Joint anatomy

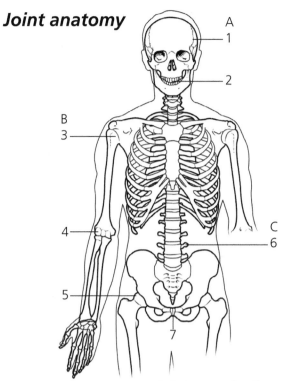

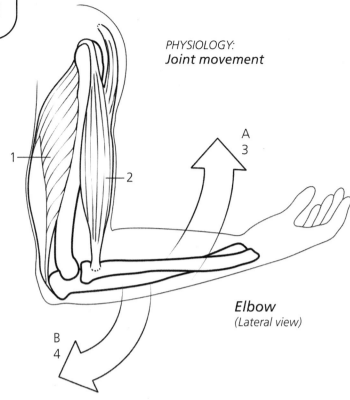

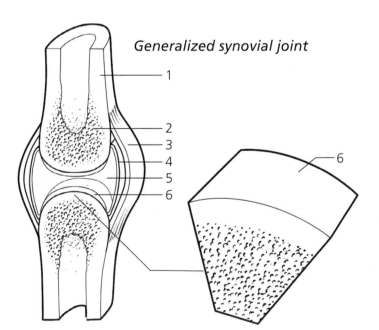

PHYSIOLOGY:
Joint movement

Elbow
(Lateral view)

Joint types by function

A – Synarthrosis (*not movable*)
- 1. Coronal suture skull
- 2. Teeth in sockets

B – Diarthrosis (*freely movable*)
- 3. Shoulder (*glenohumeral*)
- 4. Elbow (*humeroulnar, humeroradial*)
- 5. Hip (*coxal*)

C – Amphiarthrosis (*slightly movable*)
- 6. Intervertebral disc articulation
- 7. Pubic symphysis

Generalized synovial joint

○ 1. Triceps brachii muscle
○ 2. Biceps brachii muscle

A – Flexion
   ○ 3. Agonist – Biceps brachii muscle
      Antagonist – Triceps brachii muscle

B – Extension
   ○ 4. Agonist – Triceps brachii muscle
      Antagonist – Biceps brachii muscle

A skeletal muscle works by contracting, exerting a pulling force through a tendon connected to bone. In flexion the biceps brachii muscle contracts and the triceps brachii muscle relaxes, moving the lower arm upward. The muscle that produces the action is called the agonist, and the opposing muscle is called the antagonist.

This movement is reversed by the action of an opposing muscle. When the lower arm is extended, the triceps brachii muscle becomes the agonist, and the biceps brachii muscle acts as the antagonist.

Cartilage
(Cross section view)

○ 1. Compact bone   ○ 4. Synovial membrane
○ 2. Spongy bone   – 5. Synovial fluid
○ 3. Joint capsule   ○ 6. Articular cartilage

5.24

The MUSCULAR System

Joint anatomy

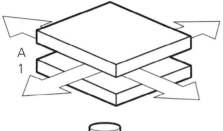

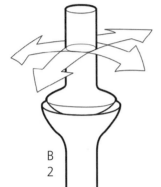

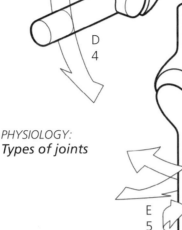

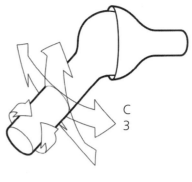

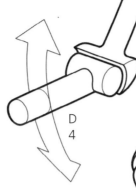

PHYSIOLOGY:
Types of joints

A – Planar or gliding
○ 1. Example: wrist

B – Ellipsoid or condylar
○ 2. Example: knuckles

C – Ball and socket
○ 3. Example: shoulder, hip

D – Hinge
○ 4. Example: elbow

E – Saddle
○ 5. Example: base of thumb

Synovial joints are divided into several main types, depending on their articular surfaces and kinds of possible movement. The hinge joint only moves in one plane, while the ball and socket joint can move along several axes. Movements of a joint can be roughly classified as circular or angular.

PHYSIOLOGY:
Muscle action – levers

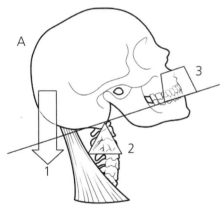

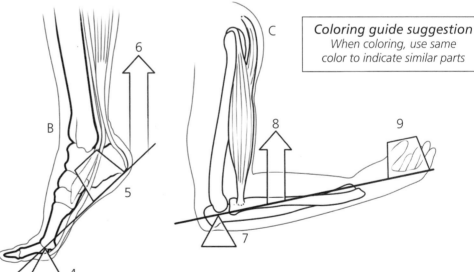

> **Coloring guide suggestion**
> *When coloring, use same color to indicate similar parts*

A – First-class lever
○ 1. Effort or force
○ 2. Fulcrum
○ 3. Weight or resistance

B – Second-class lever
○ 5. Weight or resistance
○ 4. Fulcrum
○ 6. Effort or force

C – Third-class lever
○ 7. Fulcrum
○ 8. Effort or force
○ 9. Weight or resistance

Levers are structures that move at a fixed point, or **fulcrum**. Effort or force is applied against a load or a weight. A lever, composed of muscle and bone at a joint, can change the direction, speed and distance of movement. Class 1 levers change the direction of the force, as in a seesaw. With Class 2 levers, a smaller force can move a larger load, but both speed and distance traveled are reduced. Direction remains the same. Class 3 levers move the weight in the same direction as the force. The gain is distance traveled and speed, but more force is required.

Key of abbreviations
m. Muscle   **t.** Tendon
l. Ligament

Joint anatomy: Shoulder

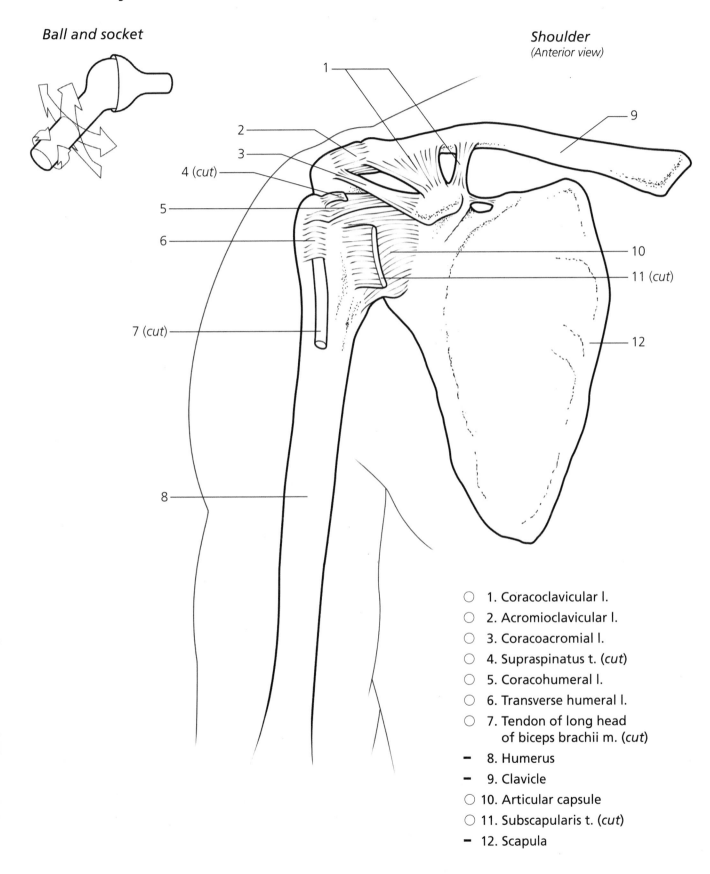

Ball and socket

Shoulder
(Anterior view)

○ 1. Coracoclavicular l.
○ 2. Acromioclavicular l.
○ 3. Coracoacromial l.
○ 4. Supraspinatus t. (*cut*)
○ 5. Coracohumeral l.
○ 6. Transverse humeral l.
○ 7. Tendon of long head
    of biceps brachii m. (*cut*)
– 8. Humerus
– 9. Clavicle
○ 10. Articular capsule
○ 11. Subscapularis t. (*cut*)
– 12. Scapula

5.26

The MUSCULAR System

Key of abbreviations
m. Muscle   **t.** Tendon
l. Ligament

Joint anatomy: Shoulder

Glenohumeral joint
(Lateral view – humerus removed)

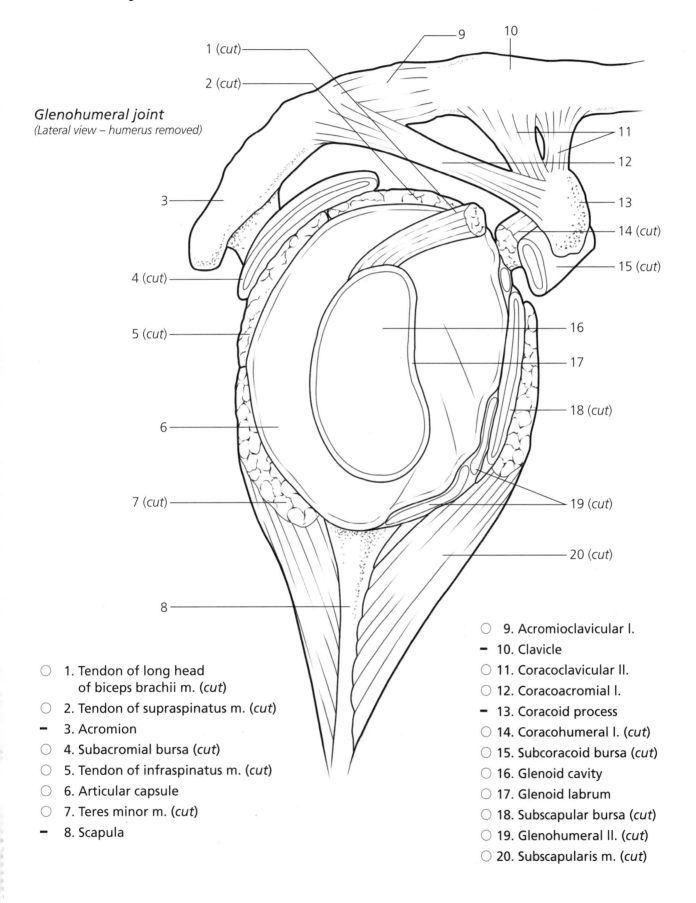

1 (*cut*)
2 (*cut*)
3
4 (*cut*)
5 (*cut*)
6
7 (*cut*)
8
9
10
11
12
13
14 (*cut*)
15 (*cut*)
16
17
18 (*cut*)
19 (*cut*)
20 (*cut*)

○ 1. Tendon of long head
   of biceps brachii m. (*cut*)
○ 2. Tendon of supraspinatus m. (*cut*)
– 3. Acromion
○ 4. Subacromial bursa (*cut*)
○ 5. Tendon of infraspinatus m. (*cut*)
○ 6. Articular capsule
○ 7. Teres minor m. (*cut*)
– 8. Scapula

○ 9. Acromioclavicular l.
– 10. Clavicle
○ 11. Coracoclavicular ll.
○ 12. Coracoacromial l.
– 13. Coracoid process
○ 14. Coracohumeral l. (*cut*)
○ 15. Subcoracoid bursa (*cut*)
○ 16. Glenoid cavity
○ 17. Glenoid labrum
○ 18. Subscapular bursa (*cut*)
○ 19. Glenohumeral ll. (*cut*)
○ 20. Subscapularis m. (*cut*)

Joint anatomy: Elbow

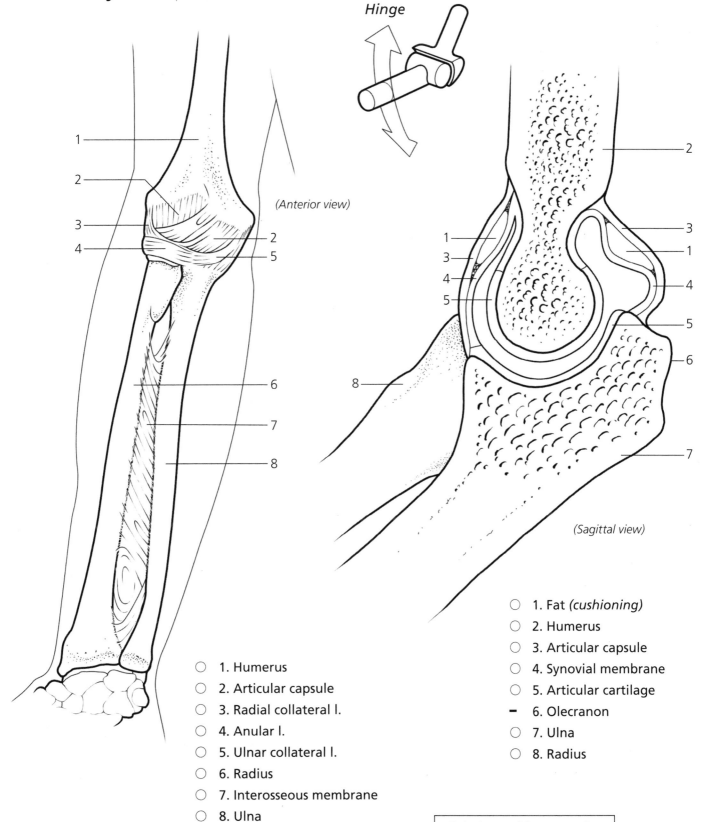

Hinge

(Anterior view)

(Sagittal view)

1. Humerus
2. Articular capsule
3. Radial collateral l.
4. Anular l.
5. Ulnar collateral l.
6. Radius
7. Interosseous membrane
8. Ulna

1. Fat (cushioning)
2. Humerus
3. Articular capsule
4. Synovial membrane
5. Articular cartilage
- 6. Olecranon
7. Ulna
8. Radius

Coloring guide suggestion
*When coloring, use same
color to indicate similar parts*

Joint anatomy: Hip

Ball and socket

(Anterior view)

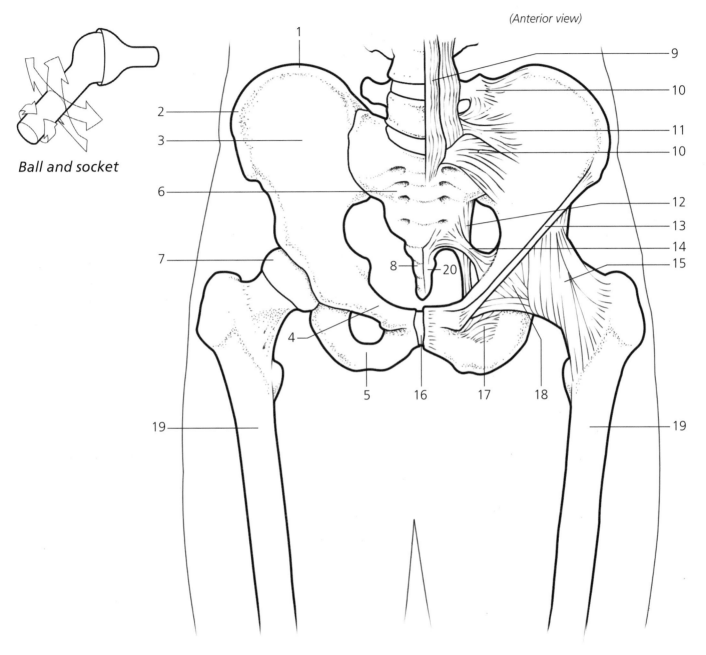

- 1. Iliac crest
- ○ 2. Os coxae
    - 3. Ilium
    - 4. Pubis
    - 5. Ischium
- ○ 6. Coccyx
- ○ 7. Head of femur
- ○ 8. Sacrum
- ○ 9. Anterior longitudinal l.
- ○ 10. Iliolumbar l.
- ○ 11. Anterior sacroiliac l.
- ○ 12. Sacrotuberous l.
- ○ 13. Inguinal l.
- ○ 14. Sacrospinous l.
- ○ 15. Iliofemoral l.
- ○ 16. Pubic symphysis
- ○ 17. Obturator membrane
- ○ 18. Pubofemoral l.
- ○ 19. Femur
- ○ 20. Anterior sacrococcygeal l.

5.29

Joint anatomy: Knee

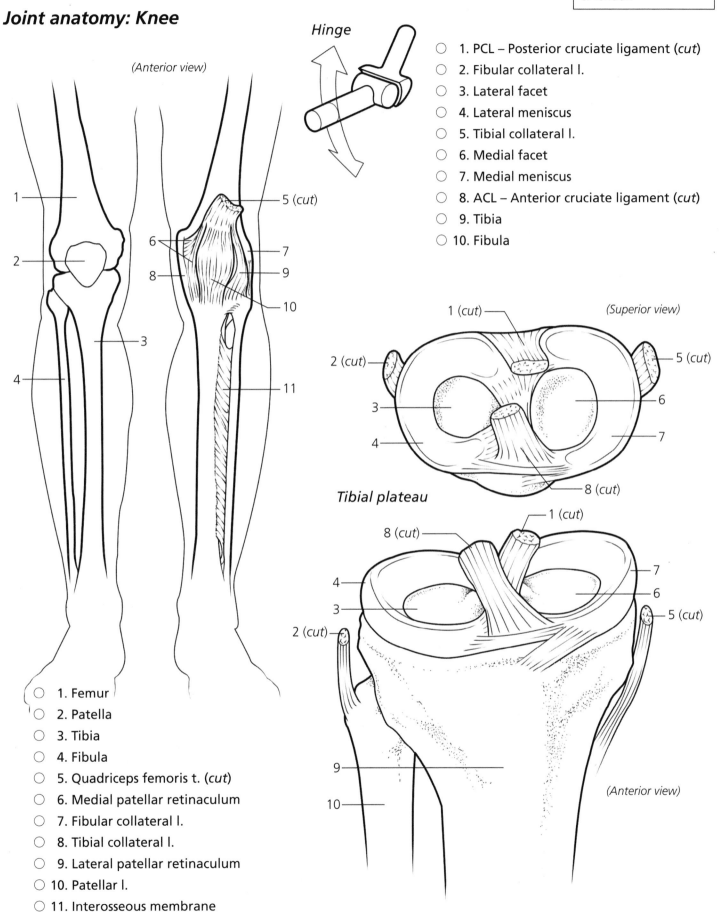

(Anterior view)

Hinge

○ 1. PCL – Posterior cruciate ligament (*cut*)
○ 2. Fibular collateral l.
○ 3. Lateral facet
○ 4. Lateral meniscus
○ 5. Tibial collateral l.
○ 6. Medial facet
○ 7. Medial meniscus
○ 8. ACL – Anterior cruciate ligament (*cut*)
○ 9. Tibia
○ 10. Fibula

(Superior view)

Tibial plateau

(Anterior view)

○ 1. Femur
○ 2. Patella
○ 3. Tibia
○ 4. Fibula
○ 5. Quadriceps femoris t. (*cut*)
○ 6. Medial patellar retinaculum
○ 7. Fibular collateral l.
○ 8. Tibial collateral l.
○ 9. Lateral patellar retinaculum
○ 10. Patellar l.
○ 11. Interosseous membrane

5.30

ANATOMY & PHYSIOLOGY COLORING BOOK

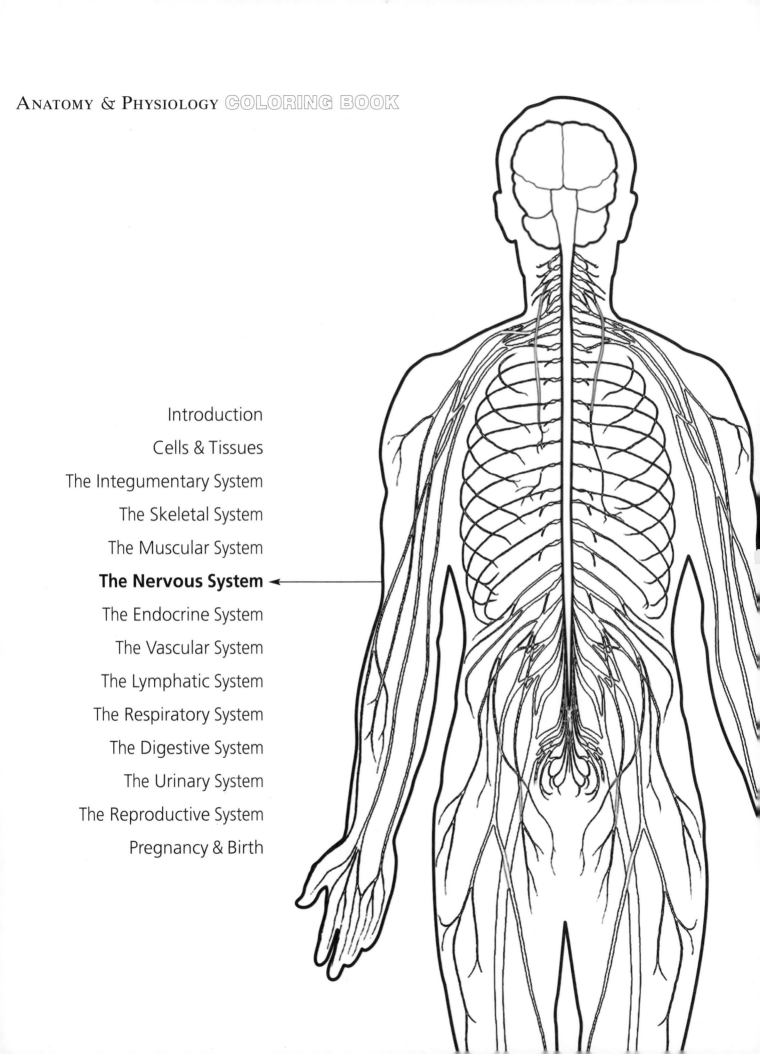

The NERVOUS System

System overview

Functional division of the Nervous System

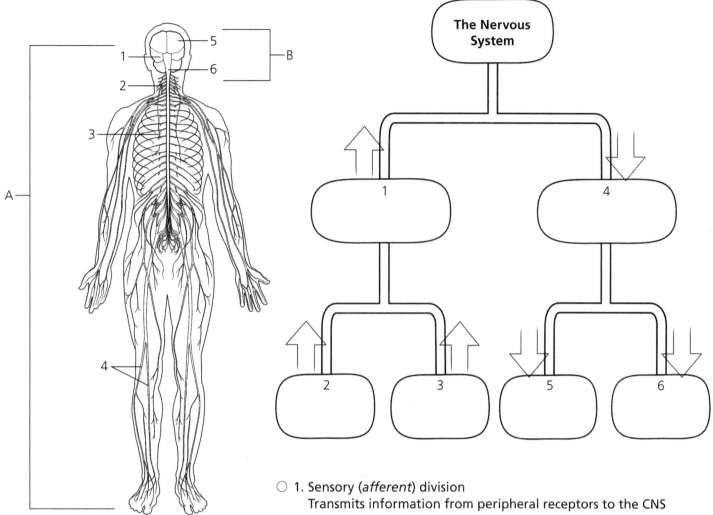

A – Peripheral nervous system (PNS)
- 1. Cranial nerves
- 2. Spinal nerves
- 3. Ganglia
- 4. Peripheral nerves

B – Central nervous system (CNS)
- ○ 5. Brain
- ○ 6. Spinal cord

○ 1. Sensory (*afferent*) division
Transmits information from peripheral receptors to the CNS

○ 2. Somatic sensory
Receives sensory inputs from skeletal muscles, joints, fascia, skin and special senses

○ 3. Visceral sensory
Receives sensory inputs from viscera (*blood vessels and organs*)

○ 4. Motor (*efferent*) division
Transmits information from the CNS to the body

○ 5. Somatic motor
"Voluntary" nervous system – skeletal muscle

○ 6. Autonomic motor
"Involuntary" nervous system – cardiac muscle, smooth muscle and glands

The nervous system is composed of two integrated subdivisions that are responsible for conducting and processing sensory and motor information: the **central nervous system** (CNS) and the **peripheral nervous system** (PNS), which connects the CNS to the rest of the body. The CNS includes the brain and spinal cord, which are covered by protective membranes called **meninges** (dura mater, arachnoid, and pia mater). The brain processes and coordinates all neural signals received from the spinal cord as well as its own nerves, such as the olfactory and optic nerves. It also performs complex mental functions such as thinking and learning.

The NERVOUS System

Major nerves: CNS, chest & abdomen

(Anterior view)

○ 1. Right cerebral hemisphere
○ 2. Cerebellum
○ 3. Spinal cord
○ 4. Lateral cord
○ 5. Medial cord
○ 6. Posterior cord
○ 7. Right phrenic nerve
○ 8. Left phrenic nerve
○ 9. Subcostal nerve
− 10. Longitudinal cerebral fissure
○ 11. Left cerebral hemisphere
− 12. Brain stem
− 13. Cervical plexus
− 14. Brachial plexus
− 15. Intercostal nerves
− 16. Lumbar plexus

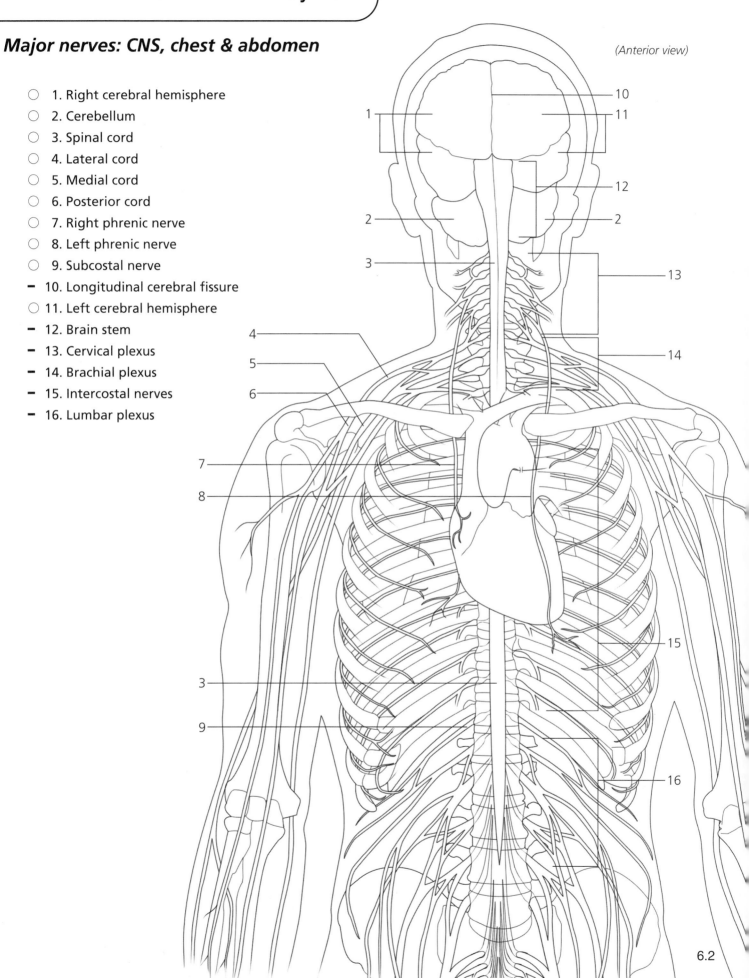

Major nerves: Arm, pelvis & lower leg

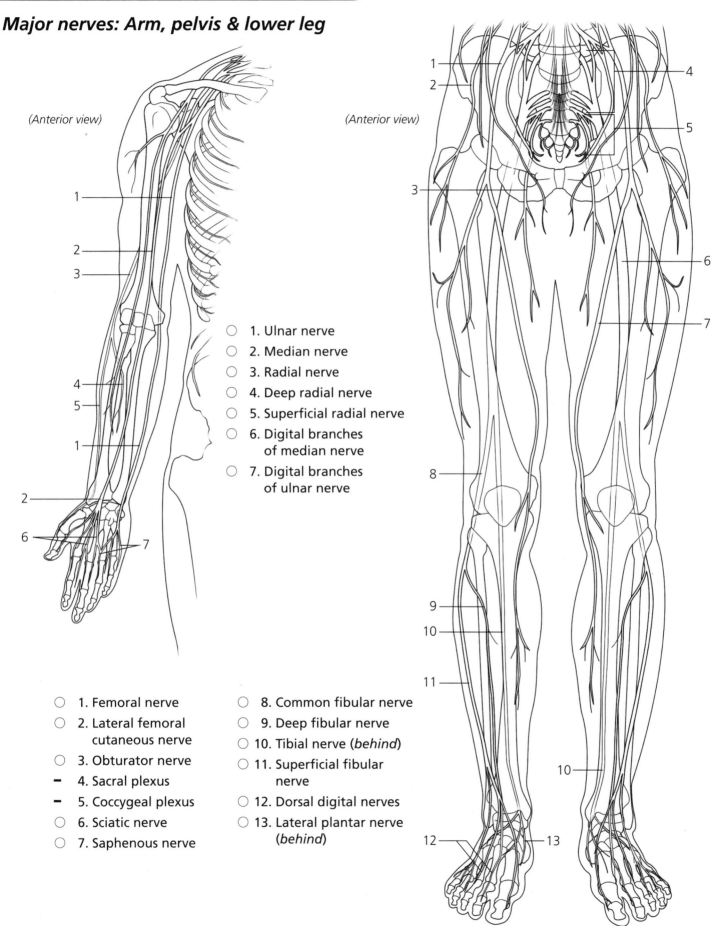

(Anterior view)

(Anterior view)

○ 1. Ulnar nerve
○ 2. Median nerve
○ 3. Radial nerve
○ 4. Deep radial nerve
○ 5. Superficial radial nerve
○ 6. Digital branches of median nerve
○ 7. Digital branches of ulnar nerve

○ 1. Femoral nerve
○ 2. Lateral femoral cutaneous nerve
○ 3. Obturator nerve
− 4. Sacral plexus
− 5. Coccygeal plexus
○ 6. Sciatic nerve
○ 7. Saphenous nerve

○ 8. Common fibular nerve
○ 9. Deep fibular nerve
○ 10. Tibial nerve (*behind*)
○ 11. Superficial fibular nerve
○ 12. Dorsal digital nerves
○ 13. Lateral plantar nerve (*behind*)

The NERVOUS System

The neuron

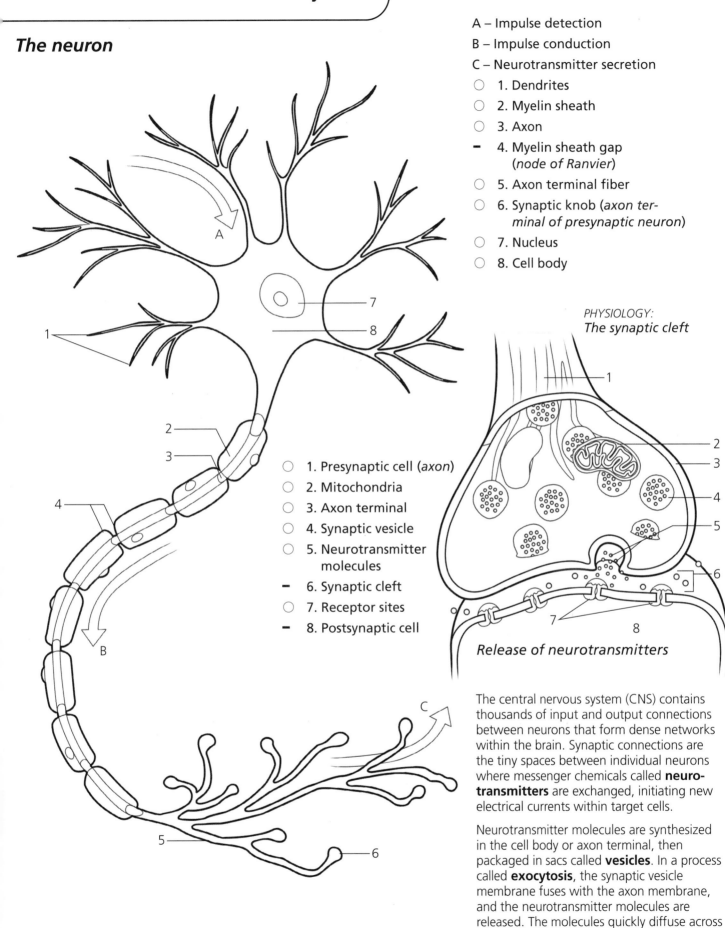

A – Impulse detection
B – Impulse conduction
C – Neurotransmitter secretion
○ 1. Dendrites
○ 2. Myelin sheath
○ 3. Axon
– 4. Myelin sheath gap
   (*node of Ranvier*)
○ 5. Axon terminal fiber
○ 6. Synaptic knob (*axon terminal of presynaptic neuron*)
○ 7. Nucleus
○ 8. Cell body

PHYSIOLOGY:
The synaptic cleft

○ 1. Presynaptic cell (*axon*)
○ 2. Mitochondria
○ 3. Axon terminal
○ 4. Synaptic vesicle
○ 5. Neurotransmitter molecules
– 6. Synaptic cleft
○ 7. Receptor sites
– 8. Postsynaptic cell

Release of neurotransmitters

The central nervous system (CNS) contains thousands of input and output connections between neurons that form dense networks within the brain. Synaptic connections are the tiny spaces between individual neurons where messenger chemicals called **neurotransmitters** are exchanged, initiating new electrical currents within target cells.

Neurotransmitter molecules are synthesized in the cell body or axon terminal, then packaged in sacs called **vesicles**. In a process called **exocytosis**, the synaptic vesicle membrane fuses with the axon membrane, and the neurotransmitter molecules are released. The molecules quickly diffuse across the synaptic cleft.

6.4

The NERVOUS System

Sensory receptor

Pressure sensor
(Lamellated disc in the skin)

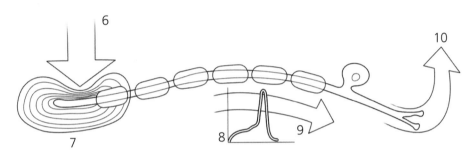

Stimulus transduction

PHYSIOLOGY:
Sensory receptor

- ○ 1. Connective tissue capsule
- ○ 2. Nerve ending
- ○ 3. Myelinated axon
- ○ 4. Nerve cell body
- ○ 5. Terminal
- ○ 6. Applied pressure
- ○ 7. Capsule deforms
- ○ 8. Generation of impulse
- ○ 9. Impulse transmission
- ○ 10. Impulse is sent to the brain

An example of a sensory receptor is the Pacinian (lamellated) corpuscle, a **mechanoreceptor** in the skin that detects pressure and vibration. The lamellations cushion the dendrite against light touch, and spread the pressure around the dendrite. The capsule deforms (mechanical), increasing permeability and depolarizing the membrane, which generates a potential (electrical). If there is enough of a stimulus, a nerve impulse is generated.

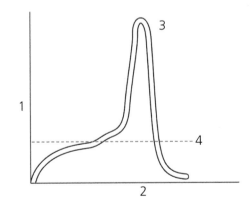

PHYSIOLOGY:
Receptor response

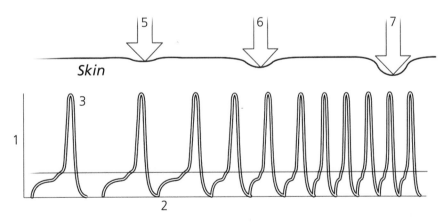

- – 1. Amplitude
- – 2. Time
- ○ 3. Nerve impulse
- – 4. Threshold potential
- ○ 5. Pressure
- ○ 6. Increasing pressure
- ○ 7. Increasing more pressure

When a stimulus is strong enough to exceed the threshold potential, a nerve impulse is generated. If the stimulus gets stronger, the **amplitude** (size and strength) of the impulse stays the same, but the rate of impulse generation increases (more pressure, more impulses).

6.5

Brain anatomy

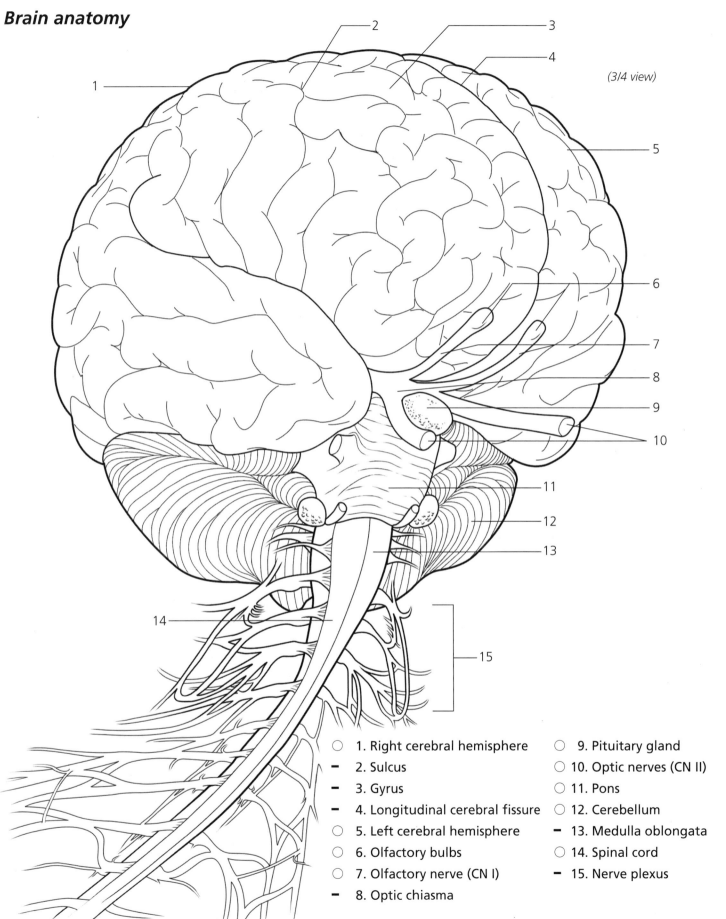

(3/4 view)

○ 1. Right cerebral hemisphere
− 2. Sulcus
− 3. Gyrus
− 4. Longitudinal cerebral fissure
○ 5. Left cerebral hemisphere
○ 6. Olfactory bulbs
○ 7. Olfactory nerve (CN I)
− 8. Optic chiasma
○ 9. Pituitary gland
○ 10. Optic nerves (CN II)
○ 11. Pons
○ 12. Cerebellum
− 13. Medulla oblongata
○ 14. Spinal cord
− 15. Nerve plexus

The NERVOUS System

Brain anatomy

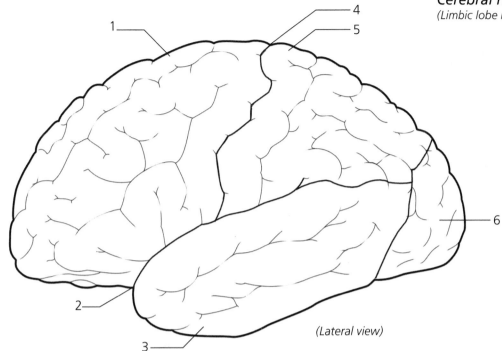

(Lateral view)

Cerebral hemisphere lobes
(Limbic lobe not shown)

- ○ 1. Frontal lobe
- – 2. Lateral sulcus
- ○ 3. Temporal lobe
- – 4. Central sulcus
- ○ 5. Parietal lobe
- ○ 6. Occipital lobe

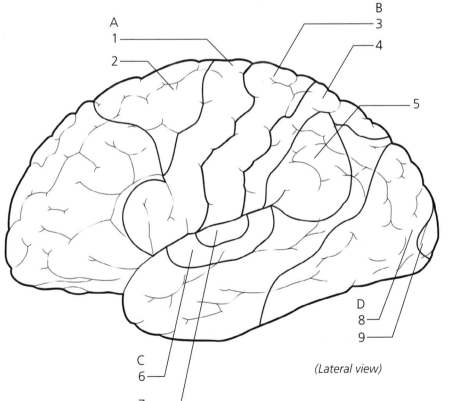

(Lateral view)

The cortex: functional areas

A – Motor function
- ○ 1. Primary area
- ○ 2. Secondary area

B – Somatosensory function
- ○ 3. Primary area
- ○ 4. Secondary area
- ○ 5. Sensory speech area
  (*Wernicke area*)

C – Acoustic auditory function
- ○ 6. Primary area
- ○ 7. Secondary area

D – Visual function
- ○ 8. Primary area
- ○ 9. Secondary area

6.7

The NERVOUS System

Brain anatomy

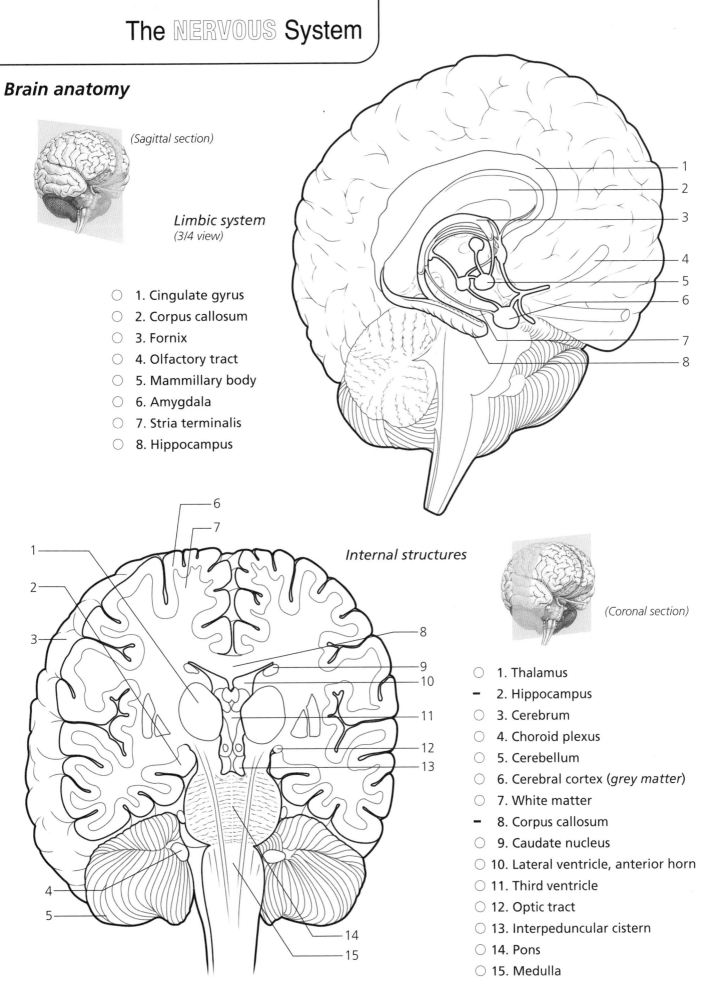

(Sagittal section)

Limbic system
(3/4 view)

○ 1. Cingulate gyrus
○ 2. Corpus callosum
○ 3. Fornix
○ 4. Olfactory tract
○ 5. Mammillary body
○ 6. Amygdala
○ 7. Stria terminalis
○ 8. Hippocampus

Internal structures

(Coronal section)

○ 1. Thalamus
− 2. Hippocampus
○ 3. Cerebrum
○ 4. Choroid plexus
○ 5. Cerebellum
○ 6. Cerebral cortex (*grey matter*)
○ 7. White matter
− 8. Corpus callosum
○ 9. Caudate nucleus
○ 10. Lateral ventricle, anterior horn
○ 11. Third ventricle
○ 12. Optic tract
○ 13. Interpeduncular cistern
○ 14. Pons
○ 15. Medulla

Brain anatomy

Ventricles
(3/4 view)

A – Lateral ventricle
- ○ 1. Anterior horn
- ○ 2. Posterior horn
- ○ 3. Inferior horn
- ○ 4. Interventricular foramen
- ○ 5. Third ventricle
- ○ 6. Cerebral aqueduct
- ○ 7. Fourth ventricle
- ─ 8. Central canal of the spinal cord

Meninges
(Sectional view)

A – Dura mater
- ○ 1. Endosteal layer
- ○ 2. Meningeal layer
- ○ 3. Arachnoid
- ○ 4. Arachnoid trabecula
- ○ 5. Artery
- ○ 6. Pia mater
- ─ 7. Cerebral cortex

The NERVOUS System

Brain anatomy

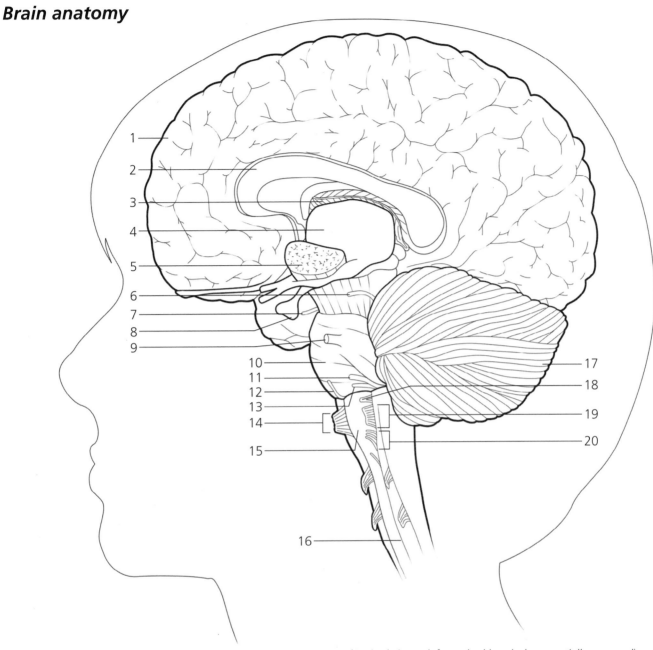

(Sagittal view – left cerebral hemisphere partially removed)

- ○ 1. Frontal cortex
- ○ 2. Corpus callosum
- ○ 3. Choroid plexus
- ○ 4. Thalamus
- ○ 5. Cerebral peduncle
- ○ 6. Trochlear nerve (CN IV)
- ○ 7. Oculomotor nerve (CN III)
- ○ 8. Pituitary gland
- ○ 9. Trigeminal nerve (CN V)
- ○ 10. Pons

- ○ 11. Facial nerve (CN VII)
- ○ 12. Abducens nerve (CN VI)
- ○ 13. Vestibulocochlear nerve (CN VIII)
- ○ 14. Hypoglossal nerve (CN XII)
- ○ 15. Medulla oblongata
- ○ 16. Spinal cord
- ○ 17. Cerebellum
- ○ 18. Glossopharyngeal nerve (CN IX)
- ○ 19. Vagus nerve (CN X)
- ○ 20. Accessory nerve (CN XI)

The NERVOUS System

Brain anatomy

(Inferior view – Nerves and spinal cord are shown cut for clarity)

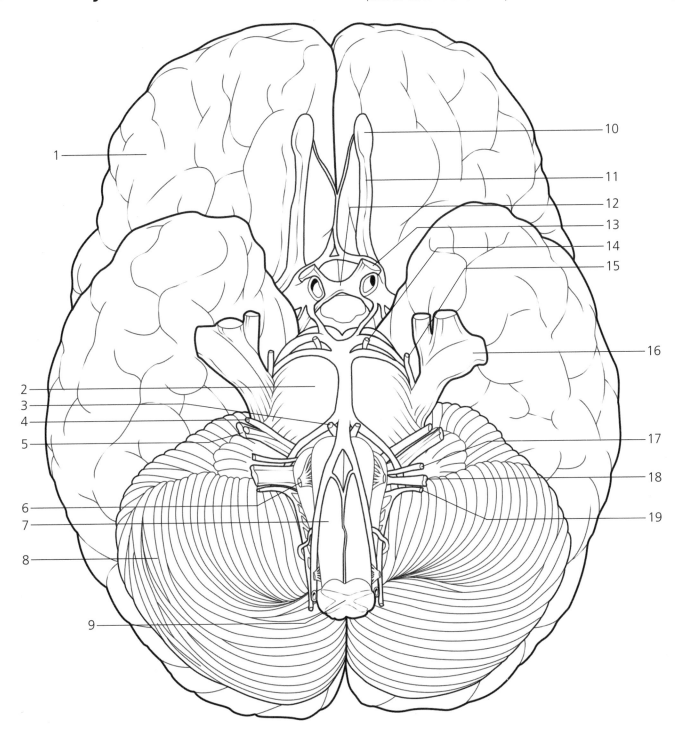

○ 1. Cerebrum

○ 2. Pons

○ 3. Abducens nerve (CN VI)

○ 4. Facial nerve (CN VII)

○ 5. Vestibulocochlear nerve (CN VIII)

○ 6. Hypoglossal nerve (CN XII)

○ 7. Medulla oblongata

○ 8. Cerebellum

○ 9. Spinal cord

○ 10. Olfactory bulb

○ 11. Olfactory nerve (CN I)

○ 12. Optic chiasm

○ 13. Optic nerve (CN II)

○ 14. Oculomotor nerve (CN III)

○ 15. Trochlear nerve (CN IV)

○ 16. Trigeminal nerve (CN V)

○ 17. Glossopharyngeal nerve (CN IX)

○ 18. Vagus nerve (CN X)

○ 19. Accessory nerve (CN XI)

Spinal cord

(3/4 view)

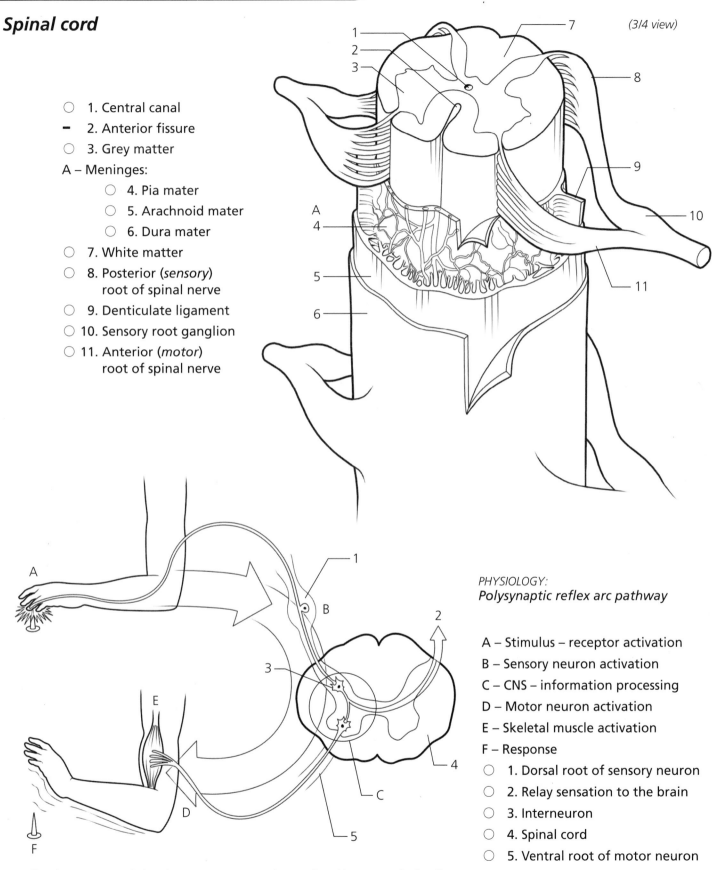

1. Central canal
2. Anterior fissure
3. Grey matter
A – Meninges:
    4. Pia mater
    5. Arachnoid mater
    6. Dura mater
7. White matter
8. Posterior (*sensory*) root of spinal nerve
9. Denticulate ligament
10. Sensory root ganglion
11. Anterior (*motor*) root of spinal nerve

PHYSIOLOGY:
Polysynaptic reflex arc pathway

A – Stimulus – receptor activation
B – Sensory neuron activation
C – CNS – information processing
D – Motor neuron activation
E – Skeletal muscle activation
F – Response
1. Dorsal root of sensory neuron
2. Relay sensation to the brain
3. Interneuron
4. Spinal cord
5. Ventral root of motor neuron

A **reflex** is an automatic involuntary response to internal and/or external stimuli. A reflex arc is a simple and quick type of nerve pathway from sensory to motor neurons. Reflexes provide protective responses to help maintain a state of balance in the body.

6.12

Brain physiology

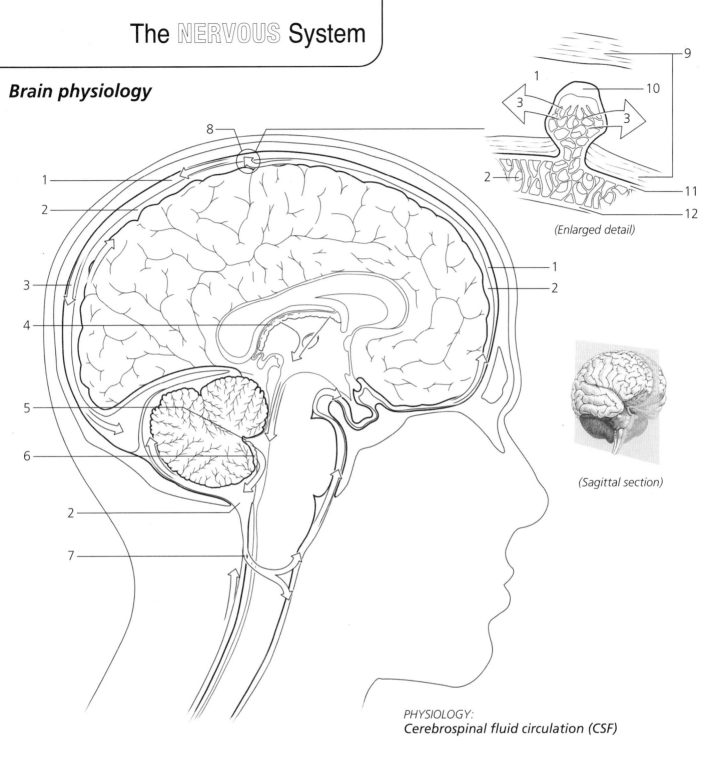

(Enlarged detail)

(Sagittal section)

PHYSIOLOGY:
Cerebrospinal fluid circulation (CSF)

- ○ 1. Superior sagittal sinus
- ○ 2. Subarachnoid space
- — 3. CSF flow
- ○ 4. Choroid plexus of third ventricle
- — 5. Lateral aperture
- ○ 6. Choroid plexus of fourth ventricle

- — 7. Median aperture
- — 8. Arachnoid villus
- ○ 9. Dura mater
- ○ 10. Arachnoid granulation
- ○ 11. Arachnoid
- ○ 12. Pia mater

Cerebrospinal fluid (CSF) is formed in the **choroid plexus**. CSF flows from the choroid plexus into the ventricles and the central canal of the spinal cord. CSF flows into subarachnoid space around the brain, finally reentering the venous system through the arachnoid granulations. Cerebrospinal fluid plays many important roles in the CNS, including acting as a shock absorber, supplying nutrients to the neurons and glial cells, transporting active biochemicals such as neurotransmitters and hormones, and removing waste products.

Brain physiology

Choroid plexus and brain capillary

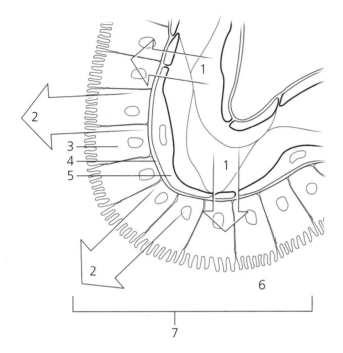

PHYSIOLOGY:
Cerebrospinal fluid formation

○ 1. Blood plasma
○ 2. Cerebrospinal fluid
○ 3. Ependymal cell
○ 4. Pia mater
○ 5. Capillary
— 6. Ventricle cavity
— 7. Choroid plexus section

Cerebrospinal fluid is mainly secreted by the **choroid plexuses**, specialized capillaries within the ventricles of the brain. CSF is a combination of an ultrafiltrate of blood and secretions of the ependymal cells lining the ventricles and central canal of the spinal cord. Cerebrospinal fluid is similar to blood plasma but contains more hydrogen, magnesium, sodium and chloride ions and less potassium and calcium ions and glucose.

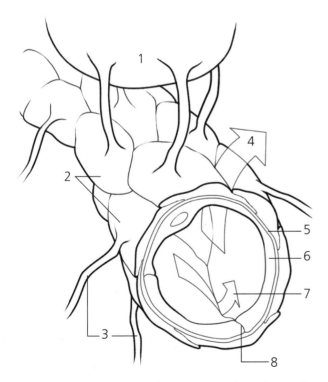

(Cross section through a capillary)

PHYSIOLOGY:
Blood-brain barrier

○ 1. Astrocyte
○ 2. Astrocyte perivascular feet
○ 3. Astrocyte dendrite process
○ 4. Nutrients (*including glucose*) and oxygen
○ 5. Continuous basement membrane
○ 6. Capillary (*endothelium*)
○ 7. Large molecules and non-lipid soluble molecules
— 8. Tight junction between endothelial cells

Hormones and other chemicals in the blood could disturb neural function, so the **blood-brain barrier** isolates neural tissue from the general circulation. The combination of tight junctions and the astrocyte covering provides reduced permeability while still allowing passage of certain substances, like oxygen and glucose.

Special senses: Sight

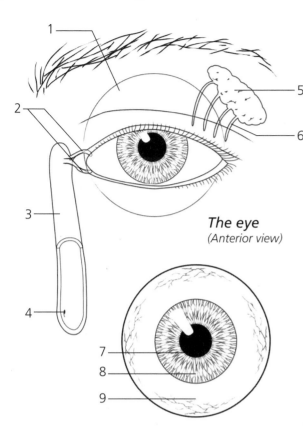

The eye
(Anterior view)

- 1. Eyeball
- ○ 2. Lacrimal canaliculi
- ○ 3. Lacrimal sac
- 4. Nasolacrimal duct
- ○ 5. Lacrimal gland
- ○ 6. Lacrimal duct
- 7. Pupil
- ○ 8. Iris
- ○ 9. Sclera (*covering*)

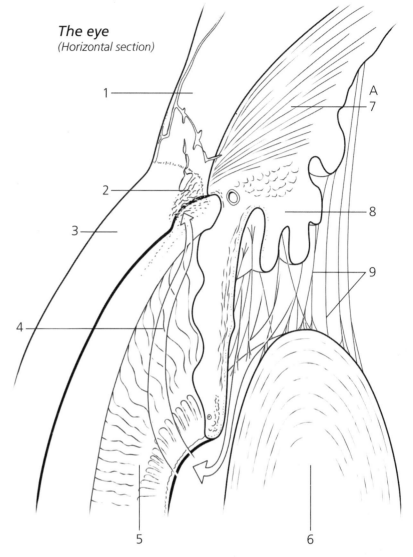

The eye
(Horizontal section)

- ○ 1. Sclera (*covering*)
- 2. Scleral venous sinus
- ○ 3. Cornea
- ○ 4. Fluid movement
- ○ 5. Iris
- ○ 6. Lens
- A – Ciliary body
  - ○ 7. Ciliary muscle
  - ○ 8. Ciliary processes
- 9. Suspensory ligaments

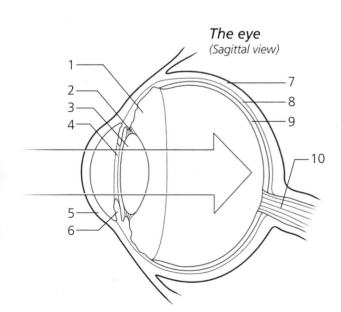

The eye
(Sagittal view)

- ○ 1. Ora serrata
- 2. Suspensory ligaments
- ○ 3. Lens
- ○ 4. Pupil
- ○ 5. Cornea
- ○ 6. Iris
- ○ 7. Sclera
- ○ 8. Choroid
- ○ 9. Retina
- ○ 10. Optic nerve

The NERVOUS System

Special senses: Sight

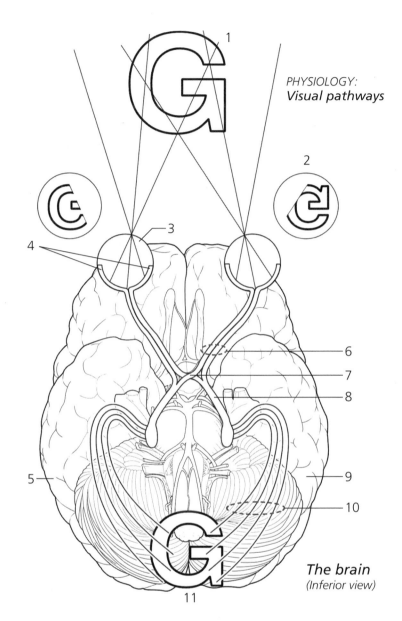

PHYSIOLOGY:
Visual pathways

The eye
(Sagittal view)

Light

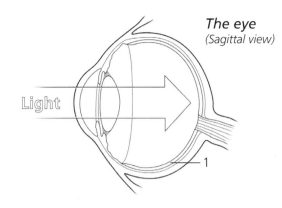

Retina
(Sagittal view)

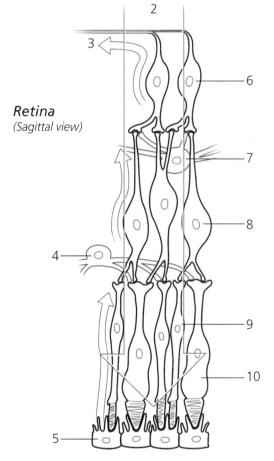

The brain
(Inferior view)

The eye

- ○ 1. External image
- ○ 2. Refracted image
- ○ 3. Eye
- ○ 4. Retina
- ○ 5. Right cerebral hemisphere
- ○ 6. Optic nerve
- – 7. Optic chiasma
- ○ 8. Optic tract
- ○ 9. Left cerebral hemisphere
- – 10. Projection fibers
- ○ 11. Processed information received in the occipital lobe

The eye

- ○ 1. Retina

Retina

- – 2. Direction of light
- ○ 3. Nerve impulse (*to optic nerve*)
- ○ 4. Horizontal cell
- ○ 5. Pigment layer
- ○ 6. Ganglion neurons
- ○ 7. Amacrine cell
- ○ 8. Bipolar cells
- ○ 9. Rod
- ○ 10. Cone

Information about the visual field travels from the retinas to the brain. Information from the right side of the visual field travels from the left halves of both retinas to the left side of the brain. The signals from the left eye cross the **optic chiasma** to reach the right side of the brain. Information about the right side of the visual field hits the right halves of both retinas and travels to the left side of the brain — the signals from the right eye also cross at the optic chiasma. Within the brain, signals travel to areas responsible for perception and eye and body movements.

Special senses: Sight

PHYSIOLOGY:
Accommodation

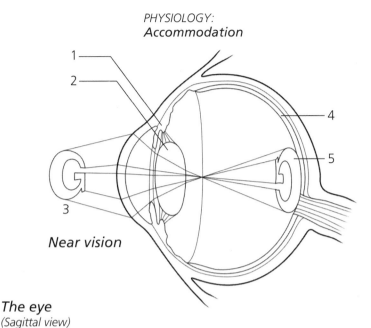

Near vision

The eye
(Sagittal view)

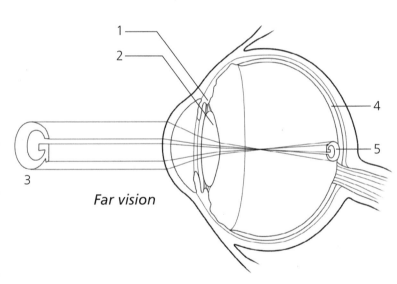

Far vision

○ 1. Ciliary body   ○ 4. Retina
○ 2. Lens   ○ 5. Refracted image
○ 3. External image

Skull
(Anterior view)

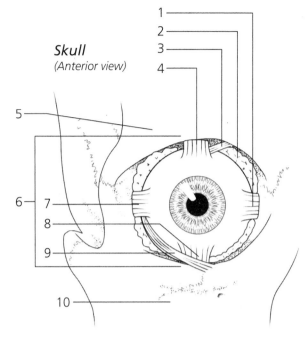

○ 1. Medial rectus m.   — 6. Orbit
○ 2. Orbital fat   ○ 7. Lateral rectus m.
○ 3. Superior oblique m.   ○ 8. Inferior rectus m.
○ 4. Superior rectus m.   ○ 9. Inferior oblique m.
— 5. Sphenoid bone   — 10. Zygomatic bone

Pupillary muscle action

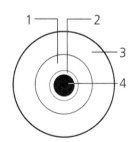

○ 1. Pupillary
    dilator muscles
○ 2. Pupillary
    constrictor muscles
○ 3. Eyeball
— 4. Pupil

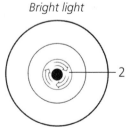

Low light

Bright light

Dilator contracts,
widening the pupil

Constrictor contracts,
narrowing the pupil

The ability of the eye to keep an image focusing on the retina is called **accommodation**. When light enters the eye, light is **refracted** or focused onto the retina. In order to keep objects that are moving in focus, the eye has to adjust this refraction. It does this by changing the shape of the lens by use of the ciliary body.

Special senses: Smell

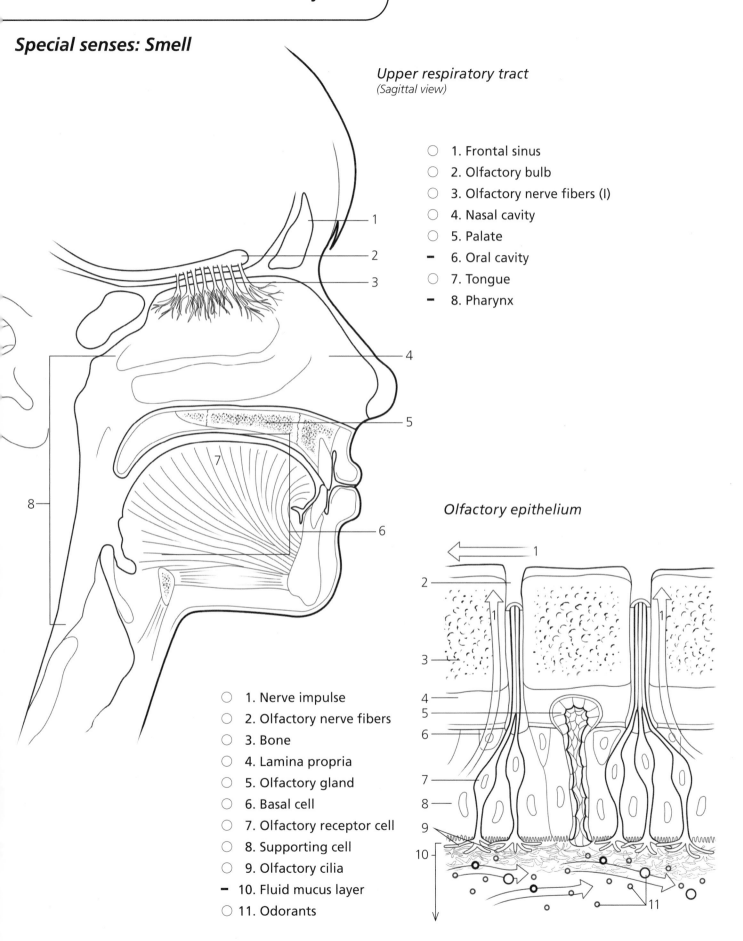

Upper respiratory tract
(Sagittal view)

○ 1. Frontal sinus
○ 2. Olfactory bulb
○ 3. Olfactory nerve fibers (I)
○ 4. Nasal cavity
○ 5. Palate
– 6. Oral cavity
○ 7. Tongue
– 8. Pharynx

Olfactory epithelium

○ 1. Nerve impulse
○ 2. Olfactory nerve fibers
○ 3. Bone
○ 4. Lamina propria
○ 5. Olfactory gland
○ 6. Basal cell
○ 7. Olfactory receptor cell
○ 8. Supporting cell
○ 9. Olfactory cilia
– 10. Fluid mucus layer
○ 11. Odorants

The NERVOUS System

Special senses: Taste

Basic tastes:
Sour   Sweet
Salty   Umami
Bitter

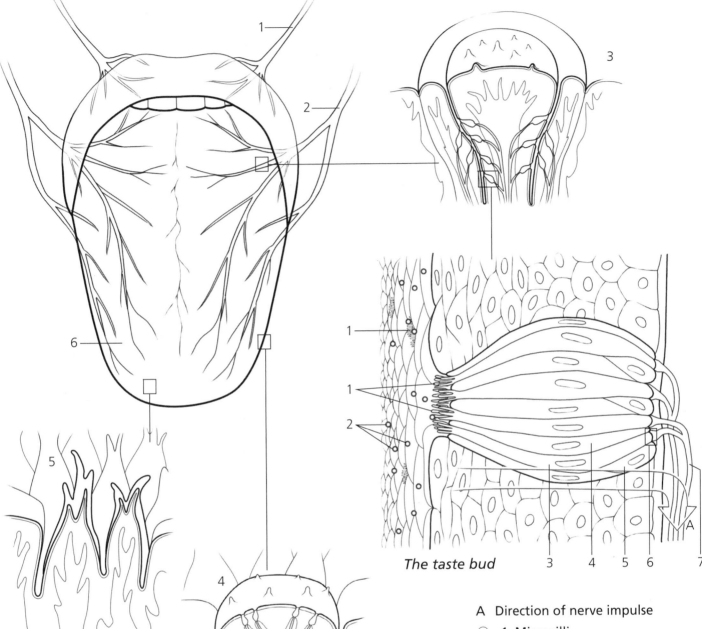

The taste bud

A   Direction of nerve impulse
○   1. Microvilli
○   2. Dissolved tastants
○   3. Gustatory cell
○   4. Supporting cell
○   5. Basal cell
−   6. Synapse
○   7. Sensory nerve

○   1. Glossopharyngeal nerve (CN IX)
○   2. Facial nerve (CN VII)
○   3. Circumvallate papilla
○   4. Fungiform papilla
○   5. Filiform papilla
−   6. Tongue

6.19

Special senses: Hearing

Outer ear

○ 1. External auditory canal
○ 2. Stapes
○ 3. Incus
○ 4. Malleus

Bones of the middle ear

○ 5. Tympanic membrane
○ 6. Tympanic cavity
○ 7. Eustachian tube
○ 8. Nasopharynx

Inner ear

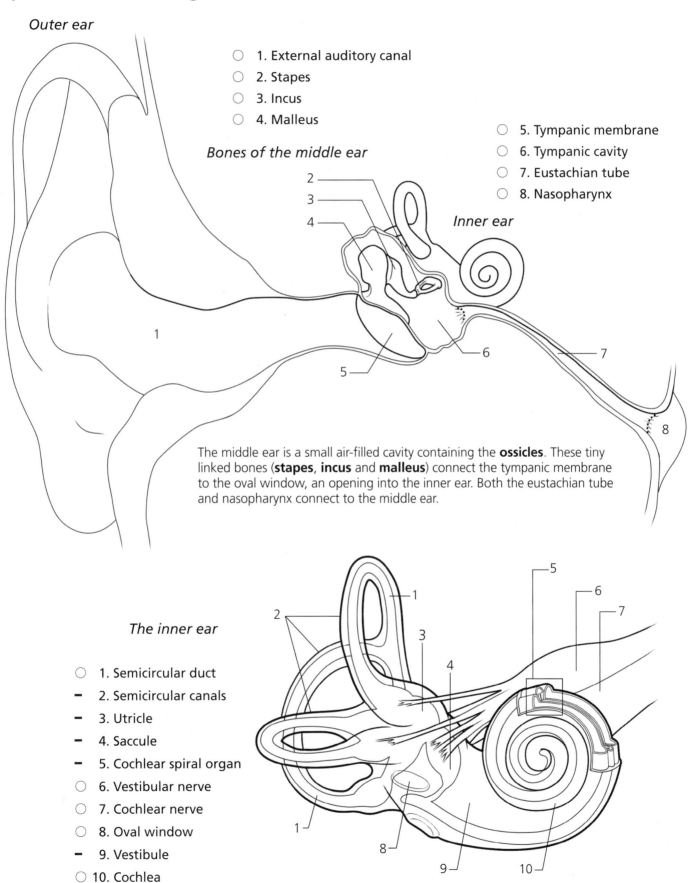

The middle ear is a small air-filled cavity containing the **ossicles**. These tiny linked bones (**stapes, incus** and **malleus**) connect the tympanic membrane to the oval window, an opening into the inner ear. Both the eustachian tube and nasopharynx connect to the middle ear.

The inner ear

○ 1. Semicircular duct
– 2. Semicircular canals
– 3. Utricle
– 4. Saccule
– 5. Cochlear spiral organ
○ 6. Vestibular nerve
○ 7. Cochlear nerve
○ 8. Oval window
– 9. Vestibule
○ 10. Cochlea

Special senses: Hearing

PHYSIOLOGY:
Sound transmission

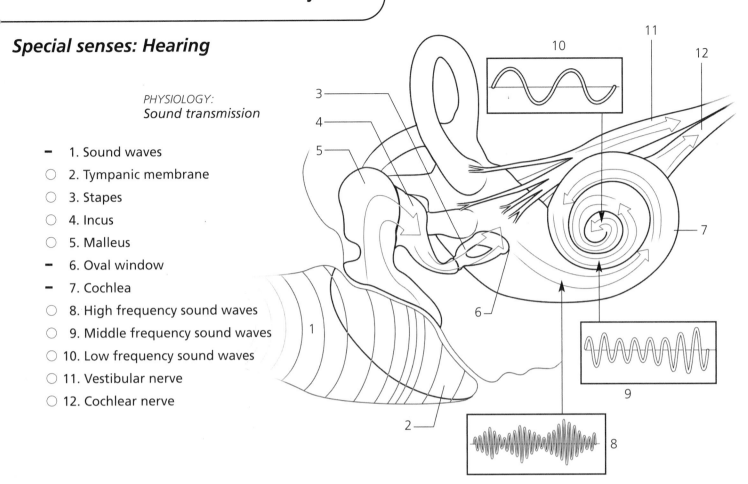

- − 1. Sound waves
- ○ 2. Tympanic membrane
- ○ 3. Stapes
- ○ 4. Incus
- ○ 5. Malleus
- − 6. Oval window
- − 7. Cochlea
- ○ 8. High frequency sound waves
- ○ 9. Middle frequency sound waves
- ○ 10. Low frequency sound waves
- ○ 11. Vestibular nerve
- ○ 12. Cochlear nerve

Airborne sound waves are collected by the external ear (**auricle**) and funneled into the auditory canal, which narrows as it approaches the tympanic membrane, amplifying the waves. The tympanic membrane vibrates in response to the sound waves and transmits vibrations to the bones of the middle ear (**ossicles**). Each of the three linked bones vibrates in a slightly different manner, intensifying the sound as the vibrations are carried across the air-filled cavity to the oval window, the entrance to the inner ear. Resulting fluid pressure waves within the inner ear stimulate receptor cells in the spiral organ in the central channel of the cochlea. Nerve impulses are carried along the cochlear nerve to the auditory center of the brain and interpreted as sound.

PHYSIOLOGY:
Sound waves

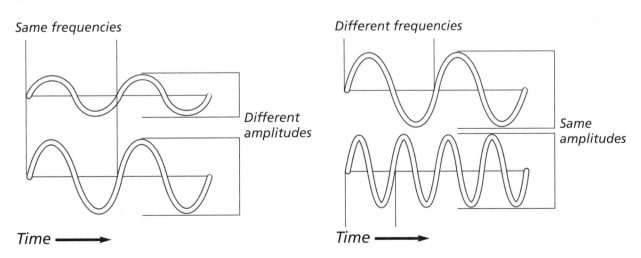

Sound waves are measured by their frequency and intensity. **Frequency** is the number of cycles per second, measured in Hertz (Hz), and it determines the pitch of a sound. **Intensity** relates to the amplitude of the sound waves and is measured in decibels (dB).

Balance

A – Macula: upright

○ 1. Macula sensors

○ 2. Nerve

○ 3. Hair cell

– 4. Otolithic membrane

○ 5. Otoliths

○ 6. Gelatinous mass

B – Macula: displaced

○ 7. Gravity

○ 8. Nerve

○ 9. Hair cell

○ 10. Gelatinous mass

○ 11. Otoliths

PHYSIOLOGY:
Balance

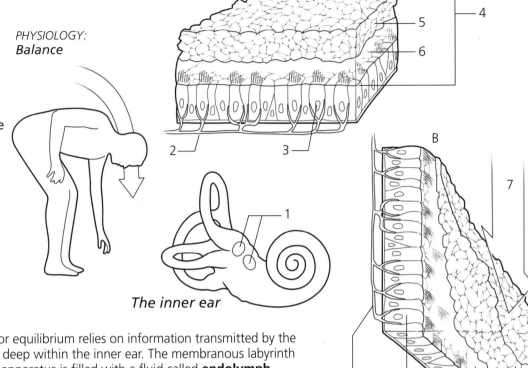

The inner ear

The body's sense of balance or equilibrium relies on information transmitted by the vestibular apparatus, located deep within the inner ear. The membranous labyrinth that makes up the vestibular apparatus is filled with a fluid called **endolymph**, which flows in response to movement of the head and body. The fluid stimulates tiny hair cells, triggering sensory neurons that relay information about position and motion to the brain.

PHYSIOLOGY:
Balance (equilibrium)

A – Crista ampullaris: stationary

– 1. Semicircular canals

○ 2. Crista ampullaris sensors

○ 3. Endolymph

○ 4. Cupula

○ 5. Hair cell (*stereocilia*)

○ 6. Nerve

B – Crista ampullaris: rotating

○ 7. Endolymph

○ 8. Centripetal force

○ 9. Cupula

○ 10. Hair cell (*stereocilia*)

○ 11. Nerve

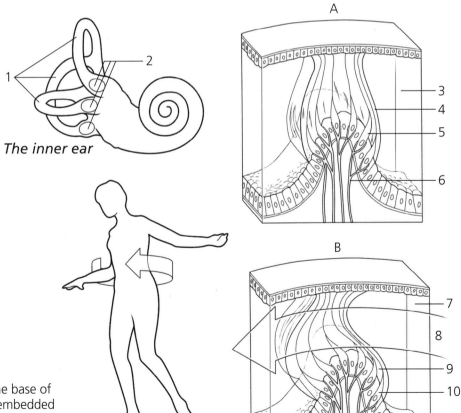

The inner ear

The crista ampullaris is in the ampulla at the base of each semicircular canal. Sensory hair cells embedded in the cone-shaped gelatinous cupula respond to fluid changes in the canal during rotational movement.

6.22

The NERVOUS System

Dermatomes

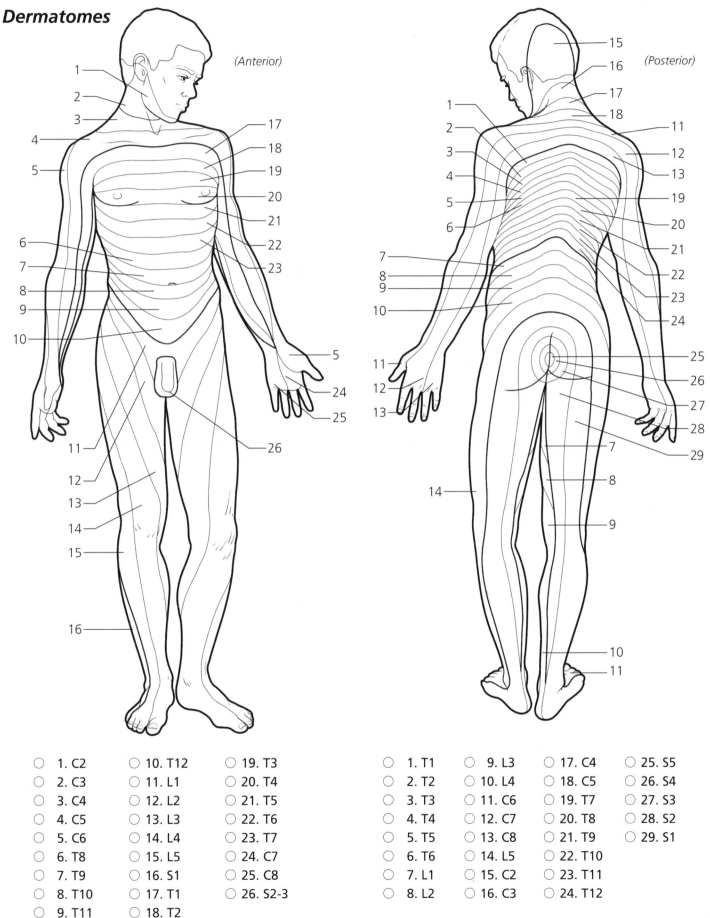

(Anterior)

(Posterior)

○ 1. C2	○ 10. T12	○ 19. T3
○ 2. C3	○ 11. L1	○ 20. T4
○ 3. C4	○ 12. L2	○ 21. T5
○ 4. C5	○ 13. L3	○ 22. T6
○ 5. C6	○ 14. L4	○ 23. T7
○ 6. T8	○ 15. L5	○ 24. C7
○ 7. T9	○ 16. S1	○ 25. C8
○ 8. T10	○ 17. T1	○ 26. S2-3
○ 9. T11	○ 18. T2	

○ 1. T1	○ 9. L3	○ 17. C4	○ 25. S5
○ 2. T2	○ 10. L4	○ 18. C5	○ 26. S4
○ 3. T3	○ 11. C6	○ 19. T7	○ 27. S3
○ 4. T4	○ 12. C7	○ 20. T8	○ 28. S2
○ 5. T5	○ 13. C8	○ 21. T9	○ 29. S1
○ 6. T6	○ 14. L5	○ 22. T10	
○ 7. L1	○ 15. C2	○ 23. T11	
○ 8. L2	○ 16. C3	○ 24. T12	

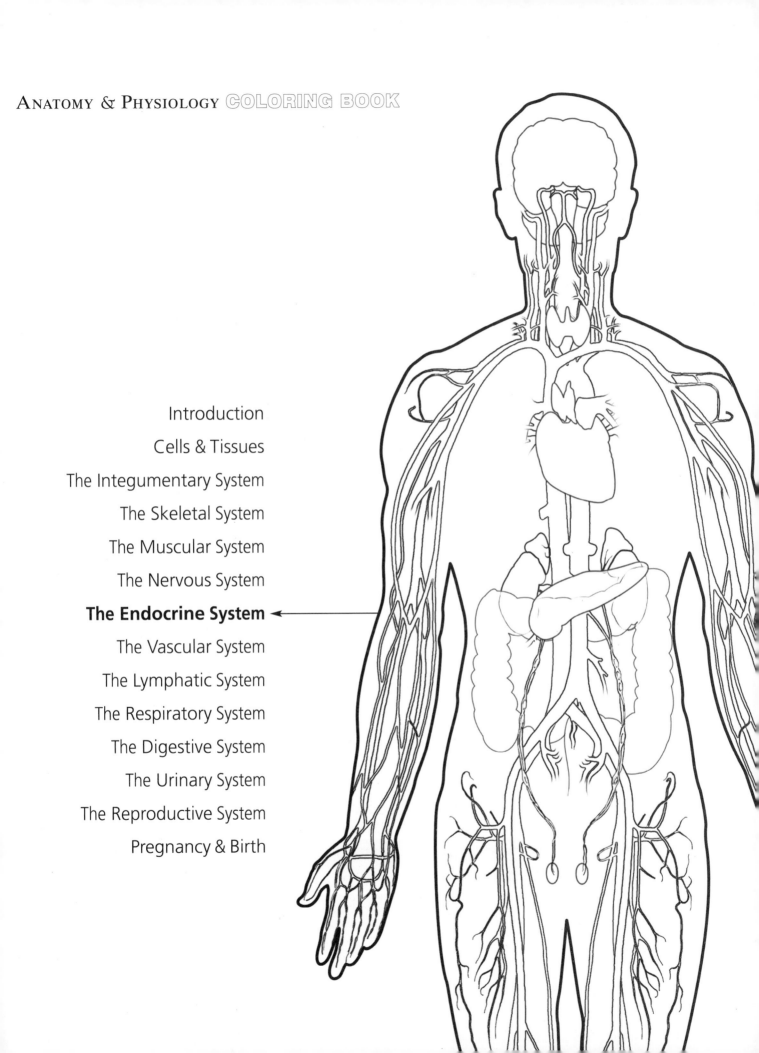

ANATOMY & PHYSIOLOGY COLORING BOOK

The ENDOCRINE System

System overview

The endocrine system is made up of dispersal organs and glands that produce **hormones**, internal chemical messengers that regulate and control functions within the body. The endocrine system regulates body processes including metabolism and energy balance, reproduction, growth and development, smooth and cardiac muscle contraction, and blood volumes of substances such as sodium and glucose. The activities of the endocrine system are closely coordinated with the nervous system.

○ 1. Thyroid and parathyroid glands
○ 2. Pancreas
− 3. Hypothalamus
− 4. Pituitary gland
− 5. Pineal gland
○ 6. Thymus
○ 7. Heart
○ 8. Adrenal gland
○ 9. Kidney
○ 10. Reproductive organs

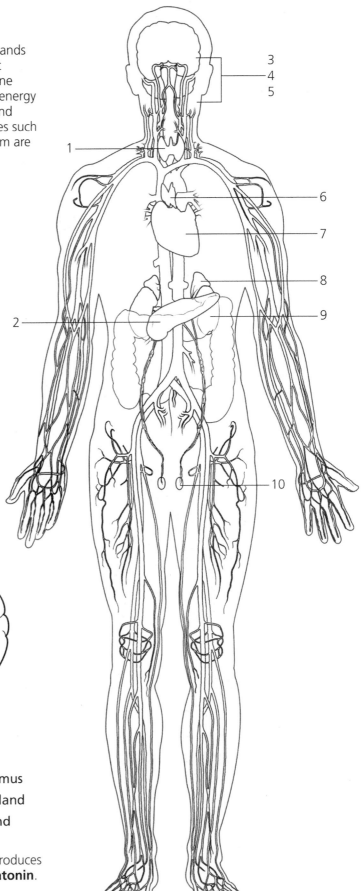

Brain
(Sagittal view)

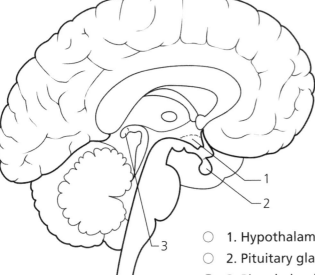

○ 1. Hypothalamus
○ 2. Pituitary gland
○ 3. Pineal gland

The pineal gland produces the hormone **melatonin**.

The ENDOCRINE System

Hormone action

PHYSIOLOGY:
Hormone action

A – Initial stimulus:
  ○ 1. From the hypothalamus
       to the pituitary gland

B – Hormone travels:
  ○ 2. From the pituitary gland
       through the vascular system
       to the target organ

○ 3. Target organ

○ 4. Hormonal response

○ 5. The level of the hormone in the
     bloodstream provides feedback
     to the pituitary gland

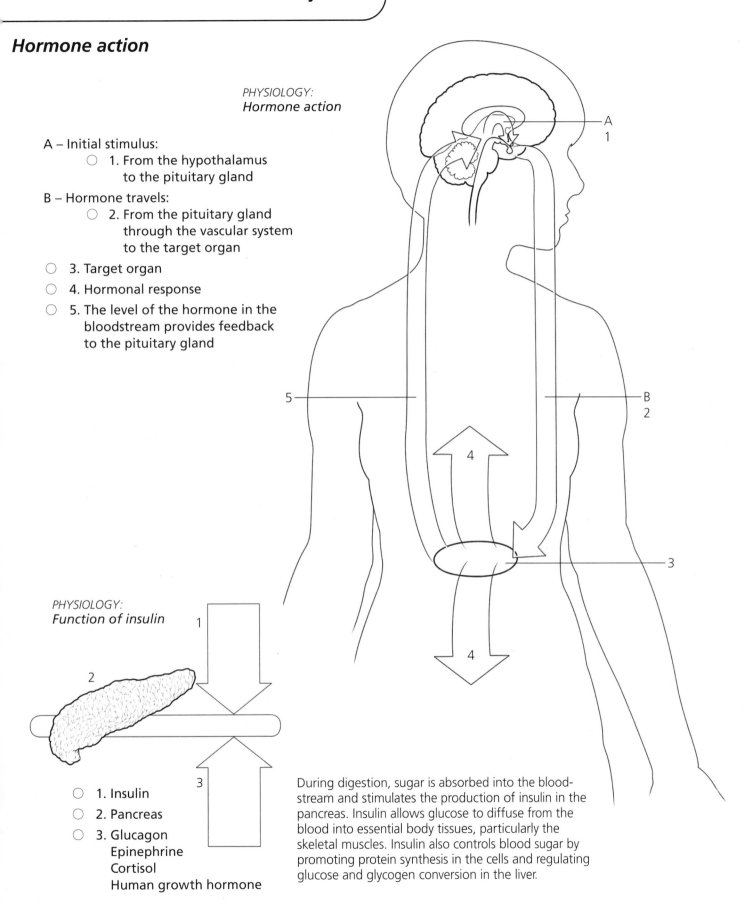

PHYSIOLOGY:
Function of insulin

○ 1. Insulin

○ 2. Pancreas

○ 3. Glucagon
     Epinephrine
     Cortisol
     Human growth hormone

During digestion, sugar is absorbed into the blood-stream and stimulates the production of insulin in the pancreas. Insulin allows glucose to diffuse from the blood into essential body tissues, particularly the skeletal muscles. Insulin also controls blood sugar by promoting protein synthesis in the cells and regulating glucose and glycogen conversion in the liver.

The ENDOCRINE System

Organs of the endocrine system

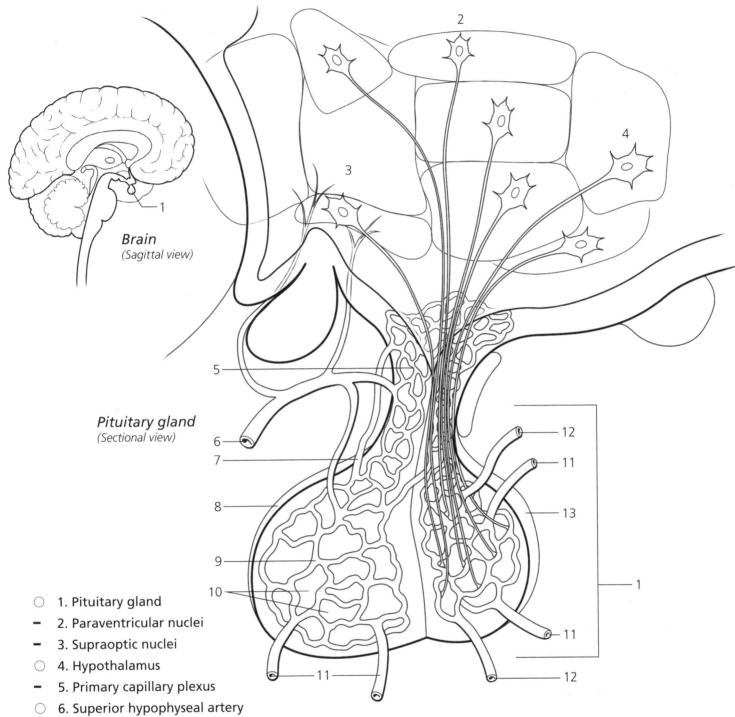

Brain
(Sagittal view)

Pituitary gland
(Sectional view)

○ 1. Pituitary gland

− 2. Paraventricular nuclei

− 3. Supraoptic nuclei

○ 4. Hypothalamus

− 5. Primary capillary plexus

○ 6. Superior hypophyseal artery

○ 7. Portal vein

− 8. Anterior lobe (*adenohypophysis*) of pituitary gland

− 9. Secondary capillary plexus

○ 10. Endocrine cells

○ 11. Branch of inferior hypophyseal vein

○ 12. Branch of inferior hypophyseal artery

− 13. Posterior lobe (*neurohypophysis*) of pituitary gland

The **pituitary gland** produces many hormones, including **growth hormone (GH)** and **antidiuretic hormone (ADH)**.

The ENDOCRINE System

Organs of the endocrine system

(Anterior views)

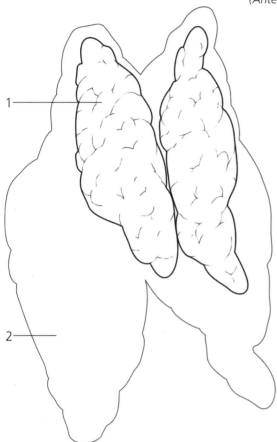

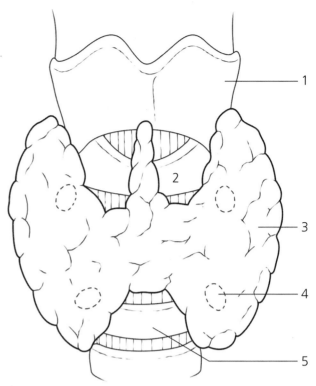

○ 1. Thyroid cartilage of larynx
○ 2. Cricoid cartilage of larynx
○ 3. Thyroid
○ 4. Parathyroid (posterior)
○ 5. Trachea

The **thyroid** and **parathyroids** produce several hormones, including **thyroxine** and **parathyroid hormone (PTH)**.

○ 1. Thymus (*adult*)
○ 2. Thymus (*juvenile*)

The **thymus** produces several hormones, including **thymosin-1** and **thymic humoral factor**. The thymus decreases in size and function (***involutes***) following puberty.

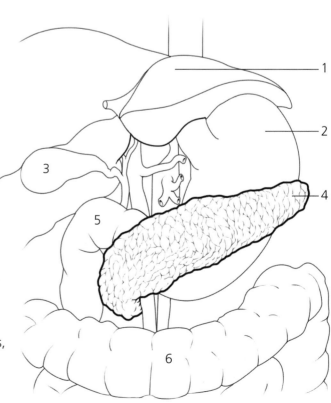

○ 1. Liver
○ 2. Stomach
○ 3. Gallbladder
○ 4. Pancreas
○ 5. Duodenum of small intestine
○ 6. Large intestine

The **pancreas** produces several hormones, including **insulin** and **glucagon**.

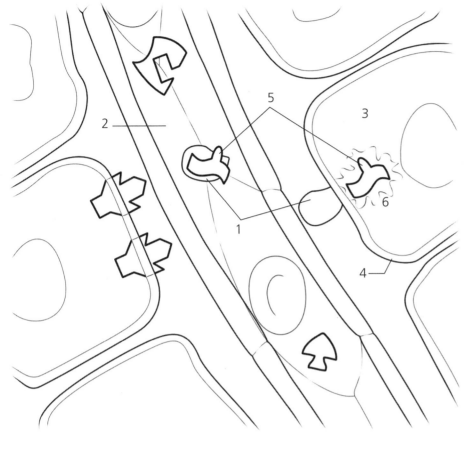

PHYSIOLOGY:
Steroid and thyroid hormones

○ 1. Protein
○ 2. Bloodstream (*capillary*)
○ 3. Target cell
○ 4. Cell membrane
○ 5. Hormone
○ 6. Cellular response

Steroid & thyroid hormones:
attach to proteins, are transported
through the bloodstream to the target
cell, and pass through the cell membrane
into the cell.

Coloring guide suggestion
When coloring, use same
color to indicate similar parts

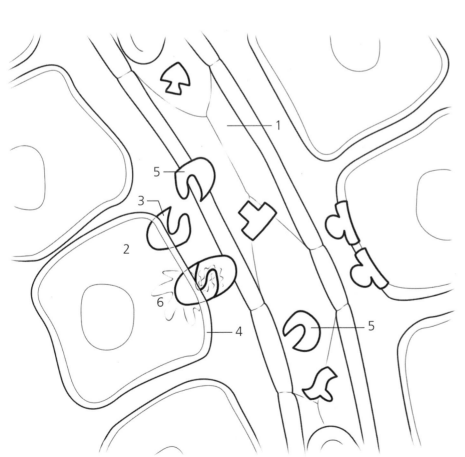

PHYSIOLOGY:
Peptide and catecholamine hormones

○ 1. Bloodstream (*capillary*)
○ 2. Target cell
○ 3. Receptor protein
○ 4. Cell membrane
○ 5. Hormone
○ 6. Cellular response

Peptide and catecholamine hormones:
travel through the bloodstream to the target
cell and bind to receptor proteins on the
cell membrane.

The ENDOCRINE System

Hormone production

(Anterior views)

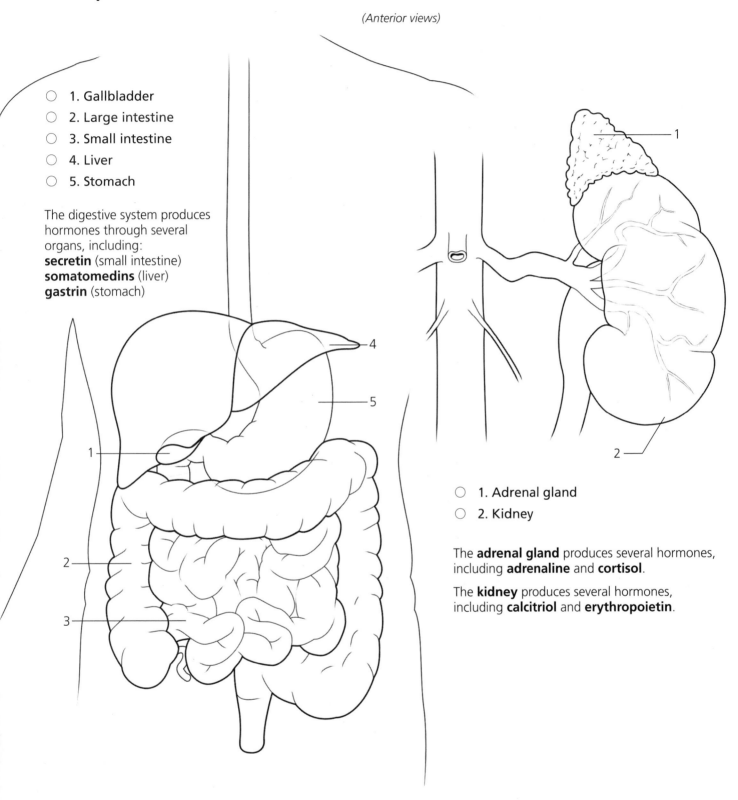

○ 1. Gallbladder
○ 2. Large intestine
○ 3. Small intestine
○ 4. Liver
○ 5. Stomach

The digestive system produces hormones through several organs, including:
secretin (small intestine)
somatomedins (liver)
gastrin (stomach)

○ 1. Adrenal gland
○ 2. Kidney

The **adrenal gland** produces several hormones, including **adrenaline** and **cortisol**.

The **kidney** produces several hormones, including **calcitriol** and **erythropoietin**.

The ENDOCRINE System

Hormone production

Female reproductive organs
(Anterior view)

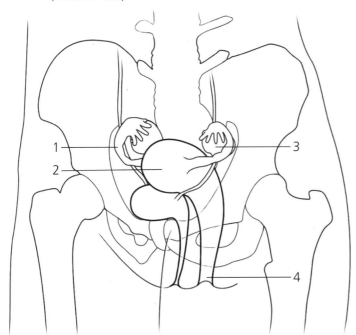

○ 1. Uterine tube
○ 2. Uterus
○ 3. Ovary
○ 4. Vagina

The **ovaries** produce several hormones, including **estradiol** and **progesterone**.

Male reproductive organs
(Anterior view)

○ 1. Seminal vesicle
○ 2. Ampulla of ductus deferens
○ 3. Prostate
○ 4. Urethra
– 5. Penis
○ 6. Ductus deferens
○ 7. Head of epididymis
○ 8. Testes
– 9. Scrotum

The **testes** produce several hormones, including **testosterone** and **inhibin**.

ANATOMY & PHYSIOLOGY COLORING BOOK

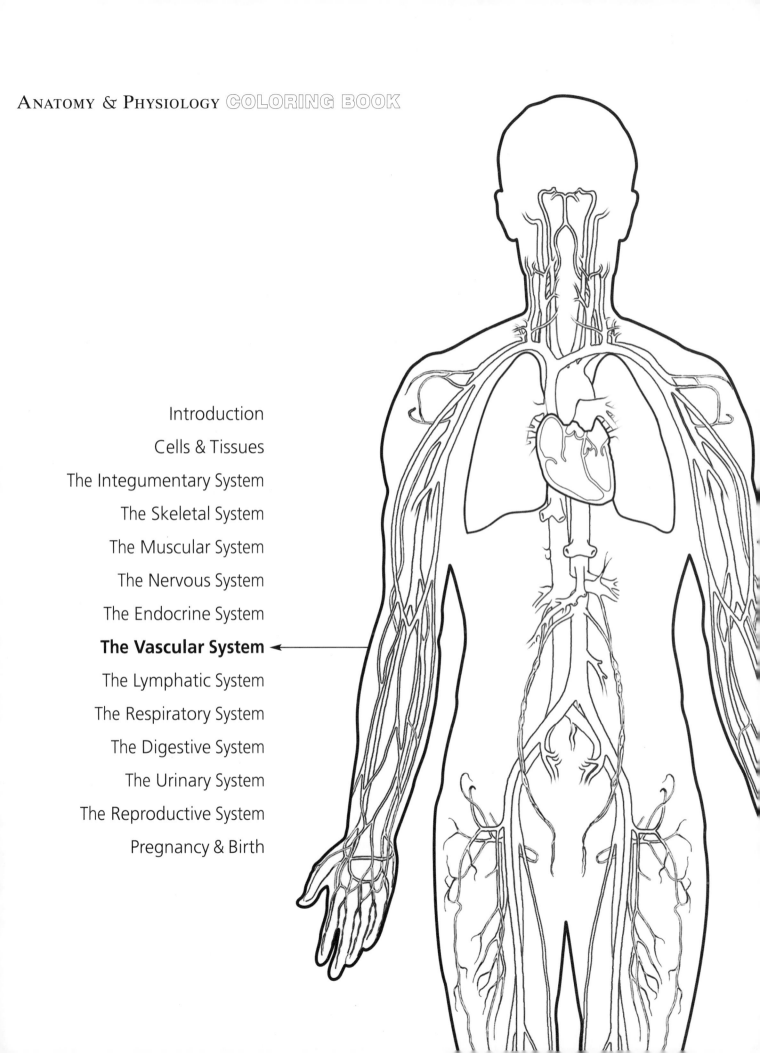

The VASCULAR System

System overview

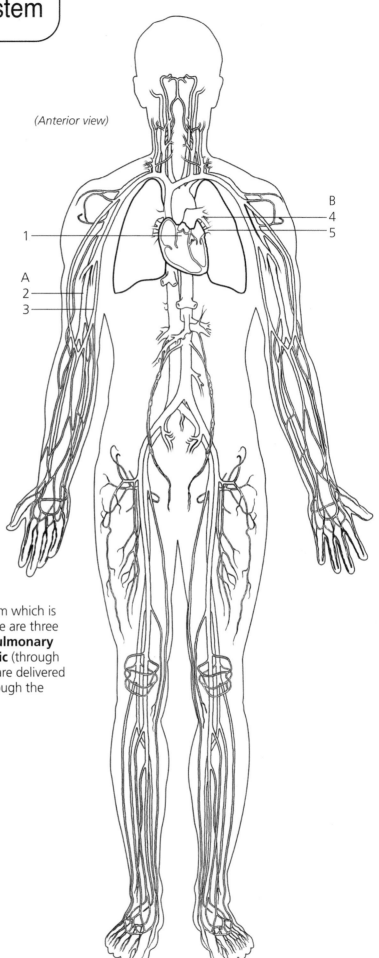

(Anterior view)

○ 1. Heart

A – Systemic circulation
   - 2. Artery
   - 3. Vein

B – Pulmonary circulation
   - 4. Pulmonary arteries
   - 5. Pulmonary veins

Every part of the body is linked by the vascular system which is made up of the heart, blood vessels and blood. There are three circulations involved: **cardiac** (through the heart), **pulmonary** (through the blood vessels in the lungs) and **systemic** (through the blood vessels in the rest of the body). Nutrients are delivered and waste products are removed from the body through the network of blood vessels in the body.

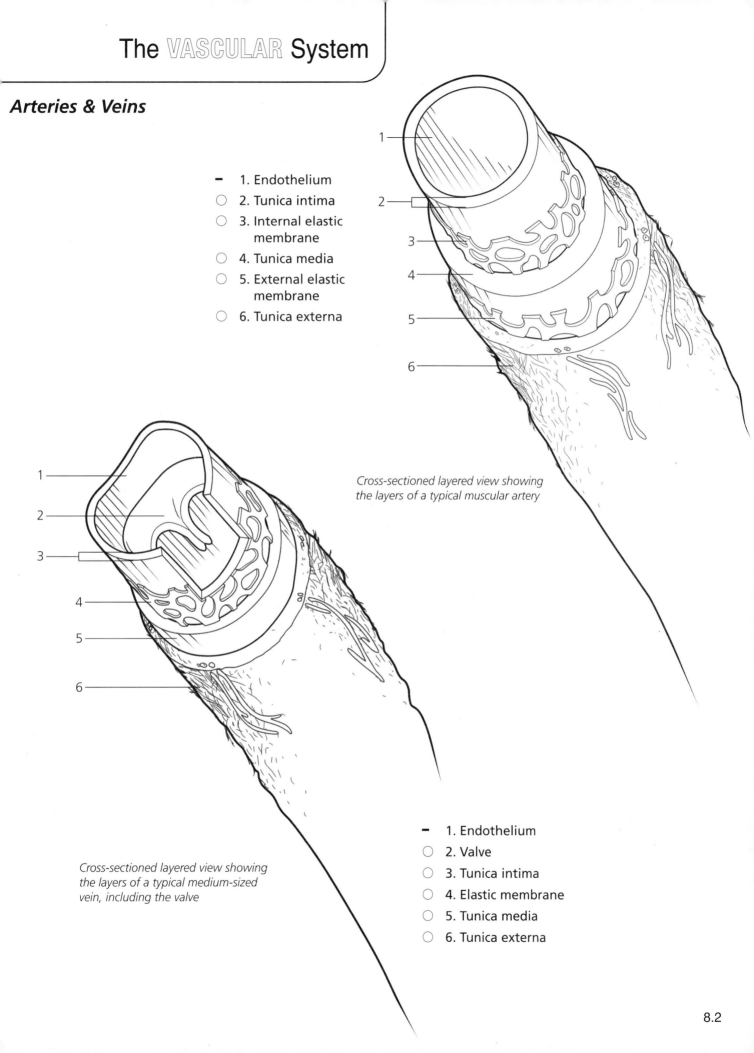

The VASCULAR System

Arteries & Veins

- 1. Endothelium
- ○ 2. Tunica intima
- ○ 3. Internal elastic membrane
- ○ 4. Tunica media
- ○ 5. External elastic membrane
- ○ 6. Tunica externa

Cross-sectioned layered view showing the layers of a typical muscular artery

Cross-sectioned layered view showing the layers of a typical medium-sized vein, including the valve

- 1. Endothelium
- ○ 2. Valve
- ○ 3. Tunica intima
- ○ 4. Elastic membrane
- ○ 5. Tunica media
- ○ 6. Tunica externa

Veins

PHYSIOLOGY:
How venous valves work

○ 1. Valve closed
○ 2. Relaxed skeletal muscles
○ 3. Vein
○ 4. Valve open
○ 5. Contracted skeletal muscles
– 6. Blood flow

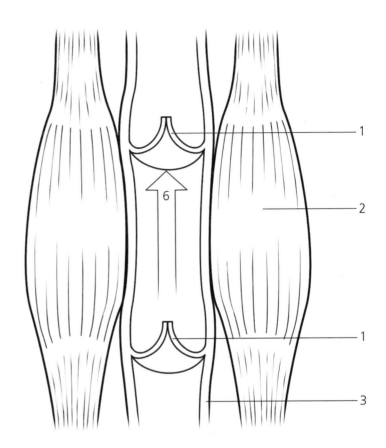

Valves inside the veins open to allow blood to flow toward the heart, and close to prevent it from flowing backward. Skeletal muscles surrounding the vein contract and compress the vein. As the upper valve opens, the lower valve remains closed, forcing the blood upward. When the muscle relaxes, the upper valve closes to prevent blood from flowing back.

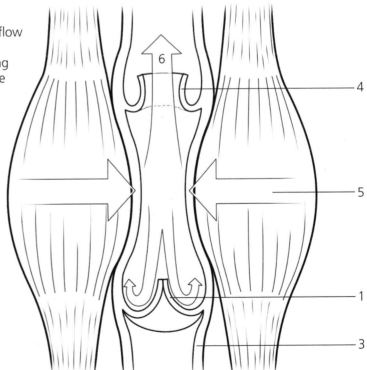

Coloring guide suggestion
When coloring, use same
color to indicate similar parts

The VASCULAR System

Blood

○ 1. Plasma:
   Water 92%
   Other 8%

○ 2. Formed elements:
   Red blood cells 99%
   White blood cells and platelets 1%

Composition of blood

Red blood cell
(cross section)

~7.5 µm

~2.6 µm

PHYSIOLOGY:
Blood cell formation

○ 1. Red bone marrow
○ 2. Hemocytoblast (*stem cell*)
○ 3. Myeloid stem cells
○ 4. Monocyte
○ 5. Red blood cells
○ 6. Platelets
○ 7. Megakaryocyte
○ 8. Basophil
○ 9. Eosinophil
○ 10. Neutrophil

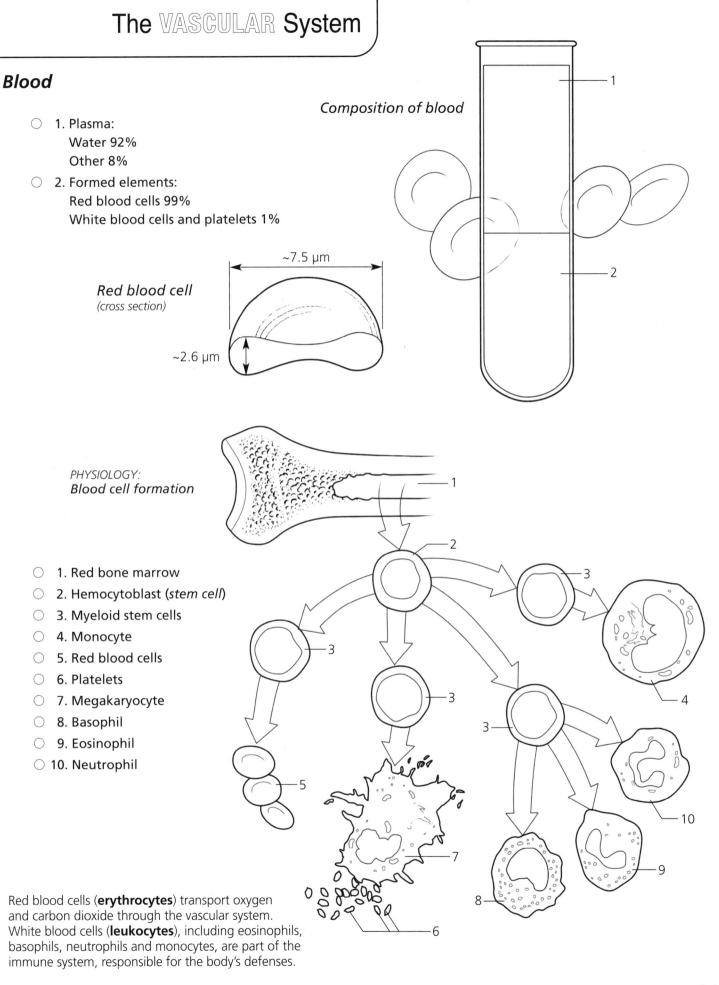

Red blood cells (**erythrocytes**) transport oxygen and carbon dioxide through the vascular system. White blood cells (**leukocytes**), including eosinophils, basophils, neutrophils and monocytes, are part of the immune system, responsible for the body's defenses.

8.4

The VASCULAR System

The heart

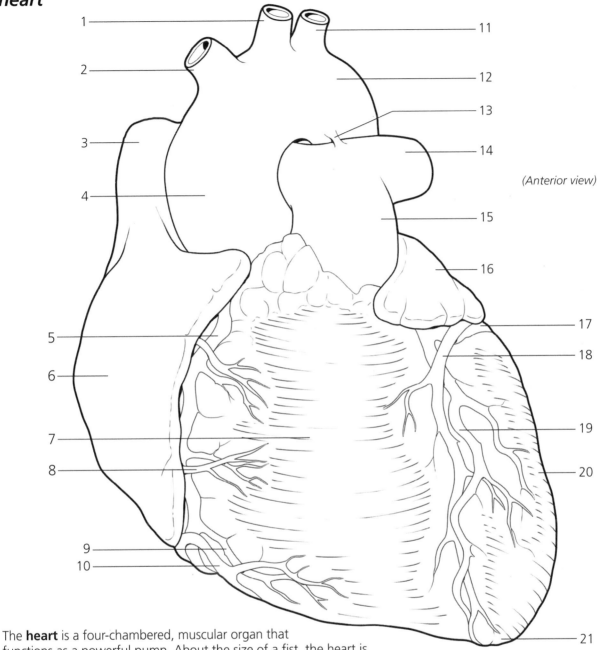

(Anterior view)

The **heart** is a four-chambered, muscular organ that
functions as a powerful pump. About the size of a fist, the heart is
located in the chest between the lungs, just to the left of center. The heart continuously pumps
blood through the body's extensive network of arteries and veins. **Arteries** transport blood away
from the heart, and **veins** transport blood back to the heart. This circulation of blood delivers oxygen
and nutrients to the body while removing waste products.

- ○ 1. Left common carotid a.
- ○ 2. Brachiocephalic a.
- ○ 3. Superior vena cava
- ○ 4. Ascending aorta
- ○ 5. Right coronary a.
- − 6. Auricle of right atrium
- − 7. Right ventricle
- ○ 8. Anterior cardiac v.

- ○ 9. Right marginal a.
- ○ 10. Small cardiac v.
- ○ 11. Left subclavian a.
- − 12. Aortic arch
- ○ 13. Ligamentum arteriosum
- ○ 14. Left pulmonary a.
- ○ 15. Pulmonary trunk
- − 16. Auricle of left atrium

- ○ 17. Circumflex a.
- ○ 18. Great cardiac v.
- ○ 19. Anterior descending (*interventricular*) a.
- − 20. Left ventricle
- − 21. Apex

The VASCULAR System

The heart

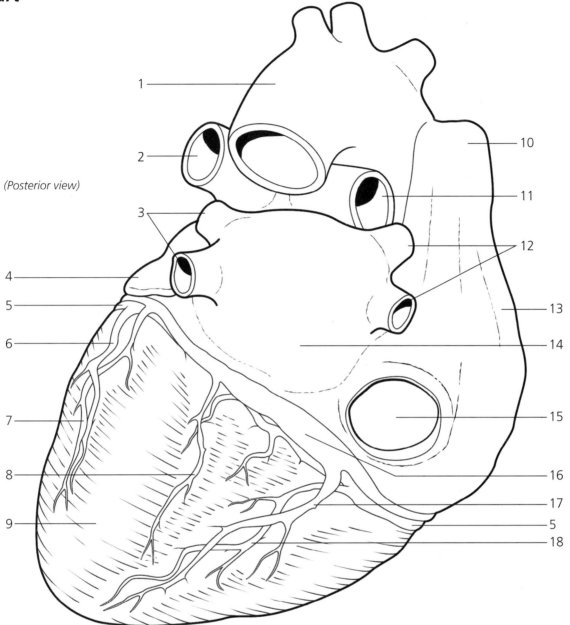

(Posterior view)

○   1. Aortic arch
○   2. Left pulmonary a.
○   3. Left pulmonary vv.
−   4. Auricle of left atrium
○   5. Circumflex a.
○   6. Left marginal a.
○   7. Left marginal v.
○   8. Left posterior ventricular v.
−   9. Left ventricle

−   10. Superior vena cava
○   11. Right pulmonary a.
○   12. Right pulmonary vv.
−   13. Right atrium
−   14. Left atrium
○   15. Inferior vena cava
○   16. Coronary sinus
○   17. Middle cardiac v.
○   18. Posterior descending (*interventricular*) a.

The VASCULAR System

The heart

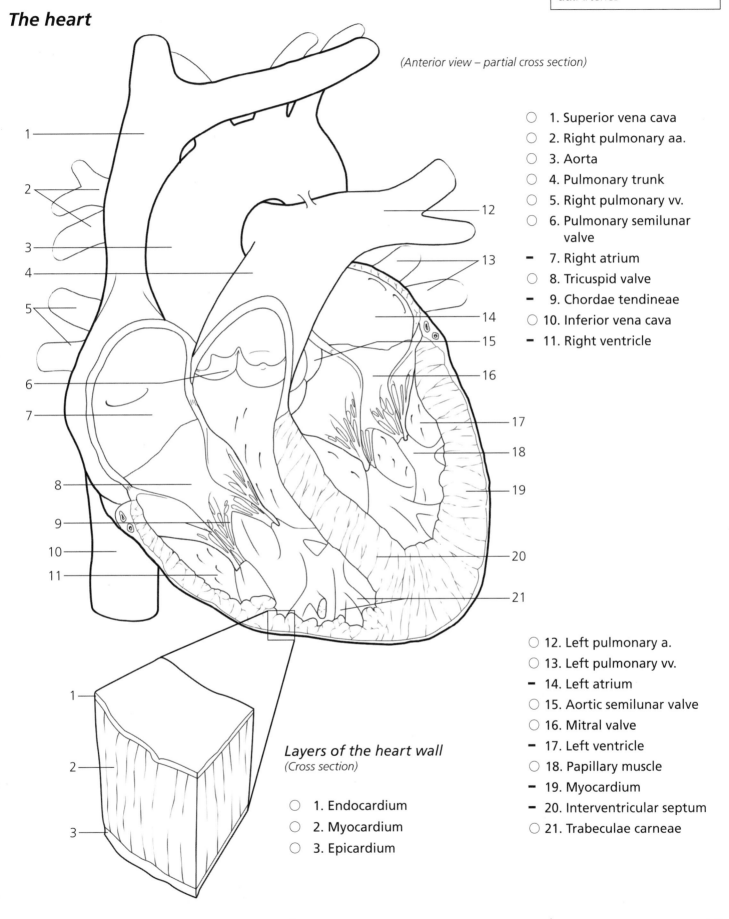

(Anterior view – partial cross section)

○ 1. Superior vena cava
○ 2. Right pulmonary aa.
○ 3. Aorta
○ 4. Pulmonary trunk
○ 5. Right pulmonary vv.
○ 6. Pulmonary semilunar valve
– 7. Right atrium
○ 8. Tricuspid valve
– 9. Chordae tendineae
○ 10. Inferior vena cava
– 11. Right ventricle

○ 12. Left pulmonary a.
○ 13. Left pulmonary vv.
– 14. Left atrium
○ 15. Aortic semilunar valve
○ 16. Mitral valve
– 17. Left ventricle
○ 18. Papillary muscle
– 19. Myocardium
– 20. Interventricular septum
○ 21. Trabeculae carneae

Layers of the heart wall
(Cross section)

○ 1. Endocardium
○ 2. Myocardium
○ 3. Epicardium

8.7

Heart valves

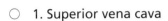

(Anterior view – partial cross section)

○ 1. Superior vena cava
○ 2. Pulmonary semilunar valve
○ 3. Tricuspid valve
○ 4. Inferior vena cava
○ 5. Right atrium
○ 6. Left atrium
○ 7. Left ventricle
○ 8. Right ventricle
○ 9. Aorta
○ 10. Left pulmonary artery
○ 11. Bicuspid valve
○ 12. Aortic semilunar valve

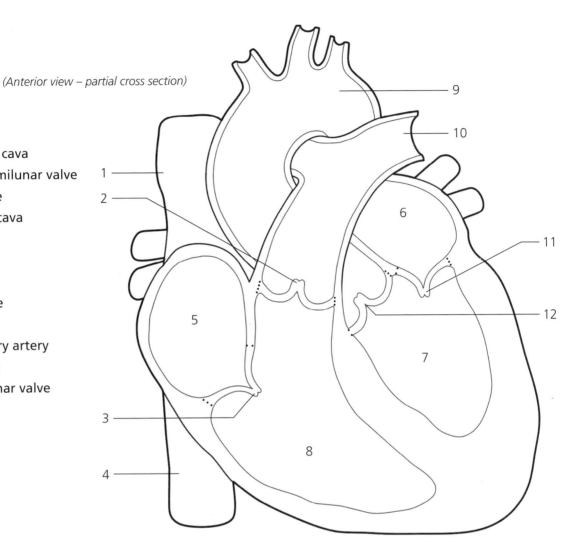

Valves
(Superior view – atria removed)

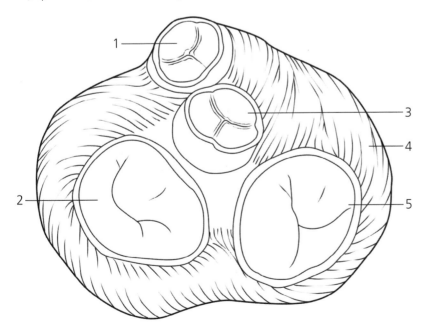

Coloring guide suggestion
*When coloring, use same
color to indicate similar parts*

○ 1. Pulmonary semilunar valve
○ 2. Bicuspid valve
○ 3. Aortic semilunar valve
○ 4. Myocardium
○ 5. Tricuspid valve

The VASCULAR System

Heart – electrical pathways

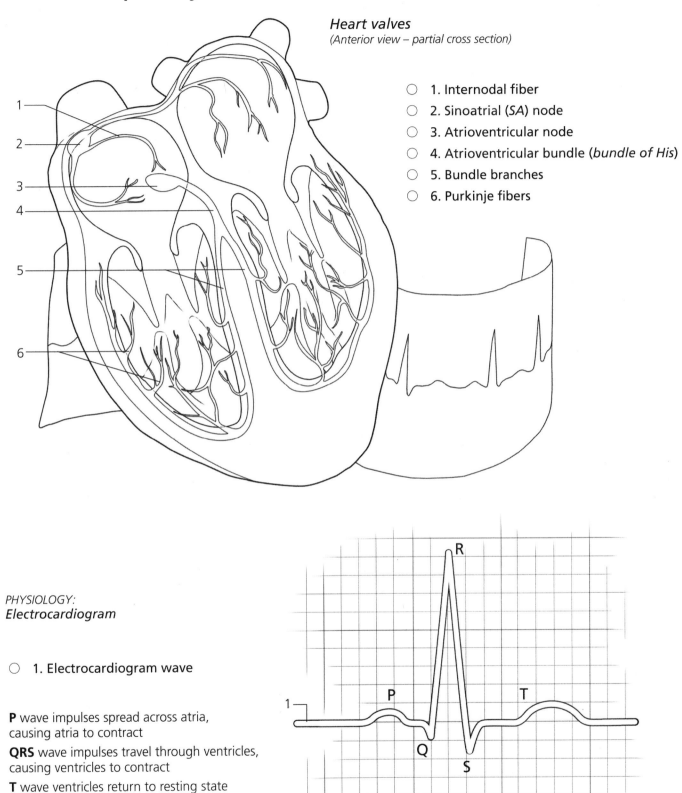

Heart valves
(Anterior view – partial cross section)

○ 1. Internodal fiber
○ 2. Sinoatrial (*SA*) node
○ 3. Atrioventricular node
○ 4. Atrioventricular bundle (*bundle of His*)
○ 5. Bundle branches
○ 6. Purkinje fibers

PHYSIOLOGY:
Electrocardiogram

○ 1. Electrocardiogram wave

P wave impulses spread across atria,
causing atria to contract

QRS wave impulses travel through ventricles,
causing ventricles to contract

T wave ventricles return to resting state

An **electrocardiogram** (ECG or EKG) graphically records the electrical activity of the heart.
A typical ECG records three waves, each representing different phases in the cardiac cycle.

PHYSIOLOGY:
Cardiac cycle

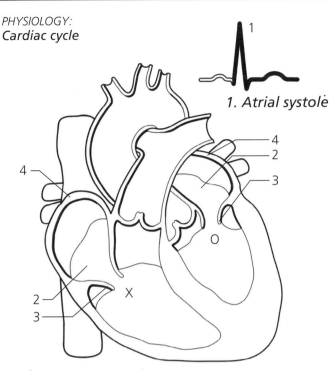

1. *Atrial systole*

○ 1. P wave
– 2. Blood returns to the heart and flows into the atria.
– 3. AV valves open; blood flows into the ventricles.
– 4. Atrial contraction

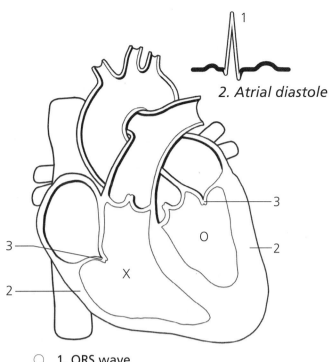

2. *Atrial diastole*

○ 1. QRS wave
– 2. Ventricles begin to contract.
– 3. AV valves close; first heart sound is heard.

> **Coloring guide suggestion**
> O - *Red* for oxygenated blood
> X - *Blue* for deoxygenated blood

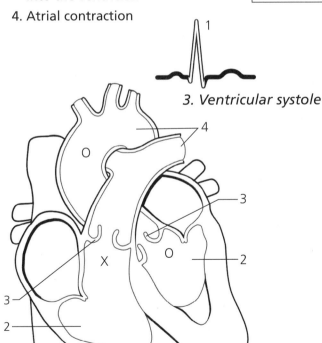

3. *Ventricular systole*

○ 1. QRS wave
– 2. Pressure rises in the ventricles.
– 3. Blood is forced out through the semilunar valves.
– 4. Blood flows into the aorta and pulmonary trunk.

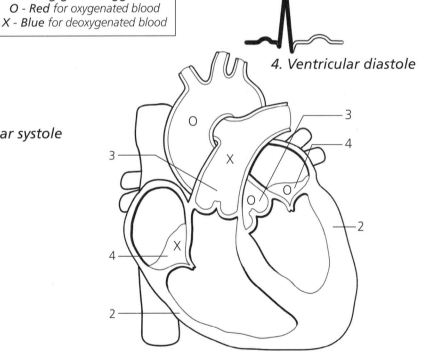

4. *Ventricular diastole*

○ 1. T wave
– 2. Ventricles relax; ventricular pressure falls.
– 3. Blood flowing back from the arteries closes the semilunar valves; second heart sound is heard.
– 4. Blood begins to fill the atria again, and the cycle repeats.

8.10

The VASCULAR System

PHYSIOLOGY:
Blood circulation

- 1. Lung
- 2. Pulmonary arteries
- 3. Heart
- ○ 4. Systemic capillaries
- ○ 5. Pulmonary capillaries
- 6. Pulmonary veins
- ○ 7. Carbon dioxide-rich blood
- ○ 8. Oxygen-rich blood

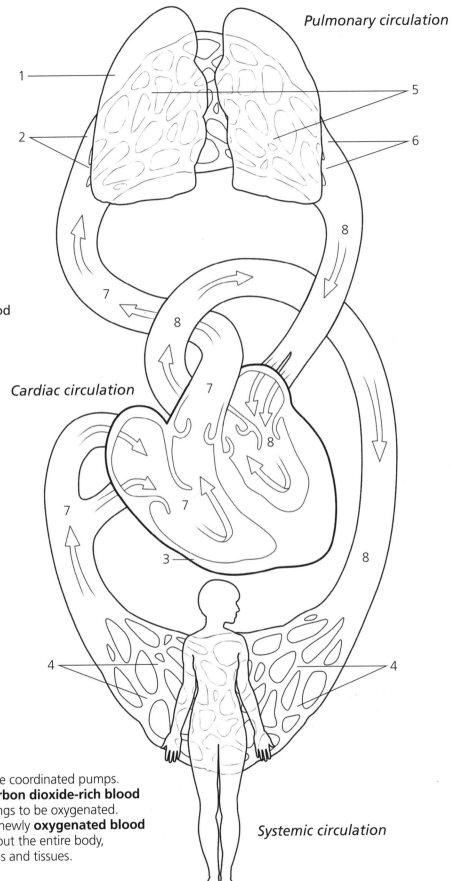

Pulmonary circulation

Cardiac circulation

Systemic circulation

The heart functions as two side-by-side coordinated pumps. The right side of the heart receives **carbon dioxide-rich blood** from the body and pumps it to the lungs to be oxygenated. The left side of the heart receives the newly **oxygenated blood** from the lungs and pumps it throughout the entire body, delivering oxygen and nutrients to cells and tissues.

The VASCULAR System

Blood pressure in different blood vessels

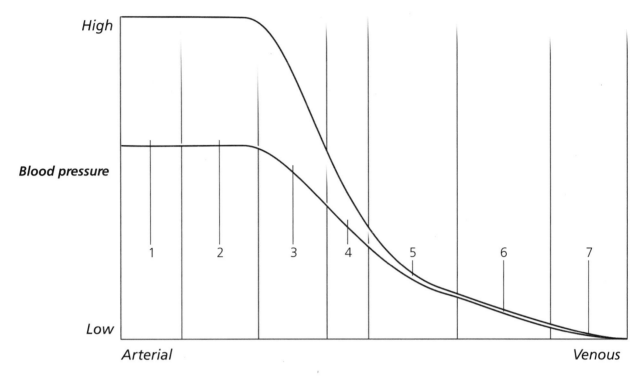

High

Blood pressure

Low

Arterial

Venous

○ 1. Aorta
○ 2. Large arteries
○ 3. Arterioles
○ 4. Precapillary sphincters

○ 5. Capillaries
○ 6. Venules
○ 7. Large veins

Blood vessels

A – Vasoconstriction
Smooth muscle contracts, narrowing the lumen or interior space, constricting blood flow.
   ○ 1. Smooth muscle contracts
   ○ 2. Lumen is narrowed

B – Vasodilation
Smooth muscle relaxes, widening the lumen or interior space, allowing blood to flow more easily.
   ○ 3. Smooth muscle relaxes
   ○ 4. Lumen is expanded

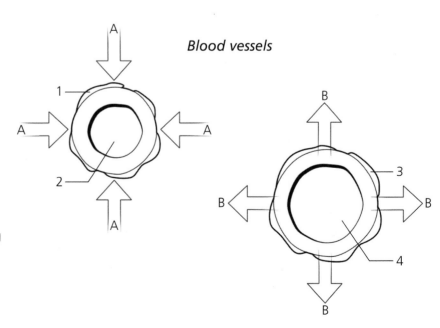

The VASCULAR System

Key of abbreviations
a. Artery
v. Vein

Vessels of the head & neck

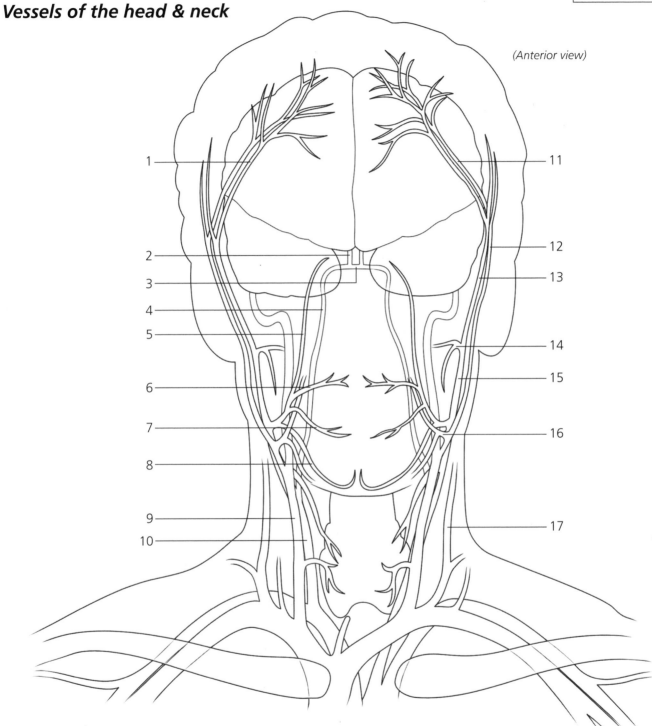

(Anterior view)

○ 1. Frontal rami of superficial temporal a.
○ 2. Anterior cerebral a.
○ 3. Anterior communicating a.
○ 4. Internal carotid a.
○ 5. Facial a.
○ 6. Superior labial a.
○ 7. Inferior labial a.
○ 8. Submental a.
○ 9. Internal jugular v.
○ 10. Common carotid a.
○ 11. Frontal rami of superficial temporal v.
○ 12. Superficial temporal v.
○ 13. Superficial temporal a.
○ 14. Maxillary a.
○ 15. External carotid a.
○ 16. Facial v.
○ 17. External jugular v.

The VASCULAR System

Arteries of the brain

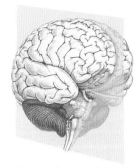

(Sagittal section)

○ 1. Paracentral a.
○ 2. Precuneal a.
○ 3. Posterior pericallosal a.
− 4. Parieto-occipital a.
○ 5. Posterior cerebral a.
− 6. Calcarine a.

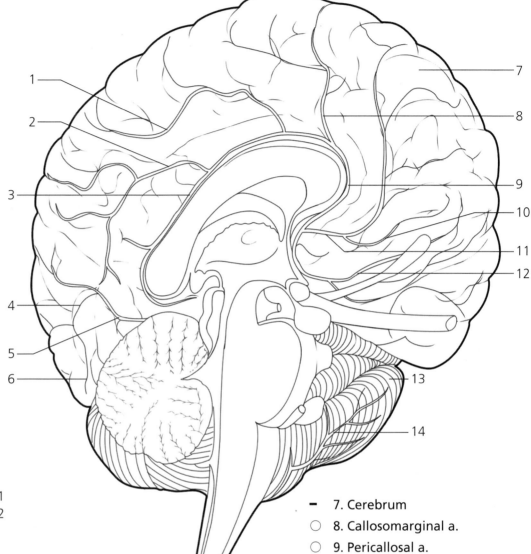

− 7. Cerebrum
○ 8. Callosomarginal a.
○ 9. Pericallosal a.
○ 10. Frontopolar a.
○ 11. Anterior cerebral a.
○ 12. Medial orbitofrontal a.
− 13. Cerebellum
○ 14. Posterior inferior cerebellar a.

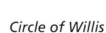

Circle of Willis
(Inferior view)

− 1. Anterior communicating a.
○ 2. Anterior cerebral a.
− 3. Internal carotid a. *(cut)*
○ 4. Middle cerebral a.
○ 5. Posterior communicating a.
○ 6. Posterior cerebral a.
○ 7. Superior cerebellar a.

− 8. Pontine aa.
○ 9. Basilar a.
○ 10. Anterior inferior cerebellar a.
○ 11. Vertebral a.
○ 12. Anterior spinal a.
○ 13. Posterior spinal a.

The VASCULAR System

Vessels of the thorax

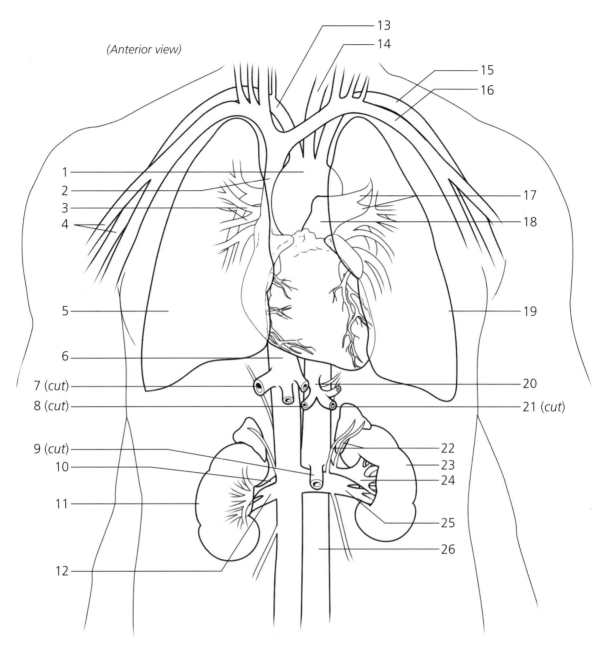

(Anterior view)

○ 1. Aortic arch
○ 2. Superior vena cava
○ 3. Right pulmonary vv.
– 4. Right axillary a. v.
– 5. Right lung
○ 6. Inferior vena cava
– 7. Hepatic veins (*cut*)
– 8. Common hepatic a. (*cut*)
– 9. Superior mesenteric a. (*cut*)

○ 10. Right renal a.
○ 11. Right kidney
○ 12. Right renal v.
○ 13. Left common carotid a.
○ 14. Brachiocephalic a.
○ 15. Left subclavian a.
○ 16. Left subclavian v.
– 17. Left pulmonary aa.
○ 18. Pulmonary trunk

– 19. Left lung
– 20. Celiac trunk
– 21. Splenic a. (*cut*)
○ 22. Left adrenal a. v.
○ 23. Left kidney
○ 24. Left renal a.
○ 25. Left renal v.
○ 26. Abdominal aorta

8.15

The VASCULAR System

Key of abbreviations
a. Artery
aa. Arteries

Digestive system arterial supply

(Anterior view – sections of several organs removed for clarity)

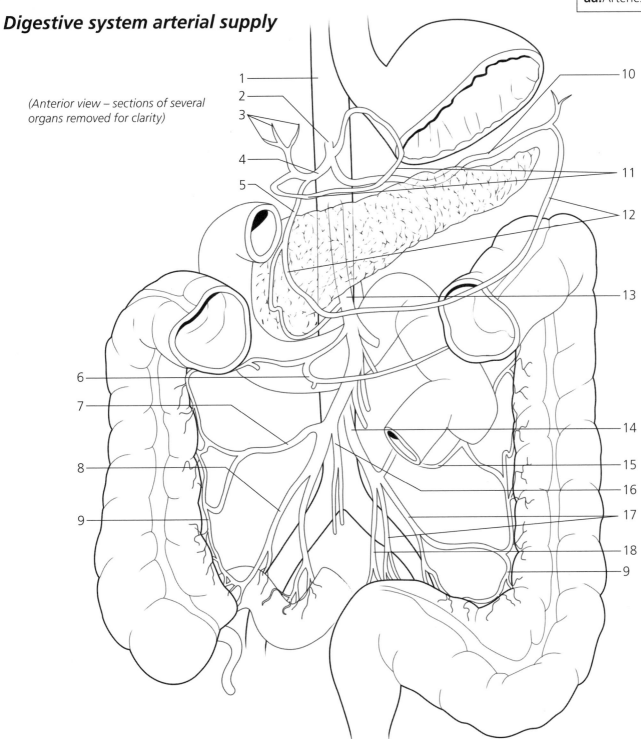

○ 1. Aorta
− 2. Celiac trunk
○ 3. Hepatic aa.
○ 4. Common hepatic a.
○ 5. Gastroduodenal a.
○ 6. Middle colic a.

○ 7. Right colic a.
○ 8. Ileocolic a.
○ 9. Marginal a.
○ 10. Splenic a.
○ 11. Gastric aa.
○ 12. Gastroepiploic aa.

○ 13. Superior mesenteric a.
○ 14. Inferior mesenteric a.
○ 15. Left colic a.
○ 16. Intestinal a.
○ 17. Sigmoid arteries
○ 18. Superior rectal a.

The VASCULAR System

Major vessels

(Anterior views)

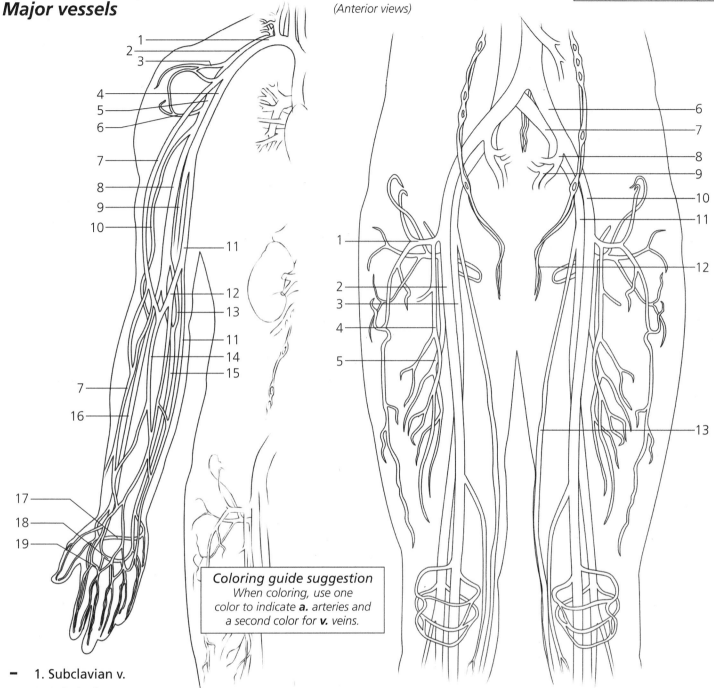

Coloring guide suggestion
*When coloring, use one color to indicate **a.** arteries and a second color for **v.** veins.*

- 1. Subclavian v.
- 2. Subclavian a.
- 3. Thoracoacromial a.
- 4. Axillary v.
- 5. Axillary a.
- 6. Anterior humeral circumflex a.
- 7. Cephalic v.
- 8. Brachial a.
- 9. Brachial v.
- 10. Deep brachial a.
- 11. Basilic v.

- 12. Median cubital v.
- 13. Anterior ulnar recurrent a.
- 14. Medial antebrachial v.
- 15. Ulnar a.
- 16. Radial a.
- ○ 17. Deep palmar arch
- ○ 18. Superficial palmar arch
- ○ 19. Superficial venous palmar arch

- 1. Lateral circumflex femoral a.
- 2. Femoral a.
- 3. Femoral v.
- 4. Deep femoral a.
- 5. Deep femoral v.
- 6. Common iliac a.
- 7. Common iliac v.

- 8. Internal iliac a.
- 9. Internal iliac v.
- 10. External iliac a.
- 11. External iliac v.
- 12. Gonadal a. v.
- 13. Saphenous v.

The VASCULAR System

Major vessels

(Anterior view)

○ 1. Descending genicular a.
– 2. Genicular a.v.
○ 3. Small saphenous v.
○ 4. Lateral tarsal a.
○ 5. Arcuate a.
○ 6. Popliteal a
○ 7. Popliteal v.
○ 8. Anterior tibial a.
○ 9. Anterior tibial v.
○ 10. Peroneal (*fibular*) a.
○ 11. Posterior tibial a.
○ 12. Posterior tibial v.
○ 13. Saphenous v.
○ 14. Dorsalis pedis a.
○ 15. Dorsal venous arch

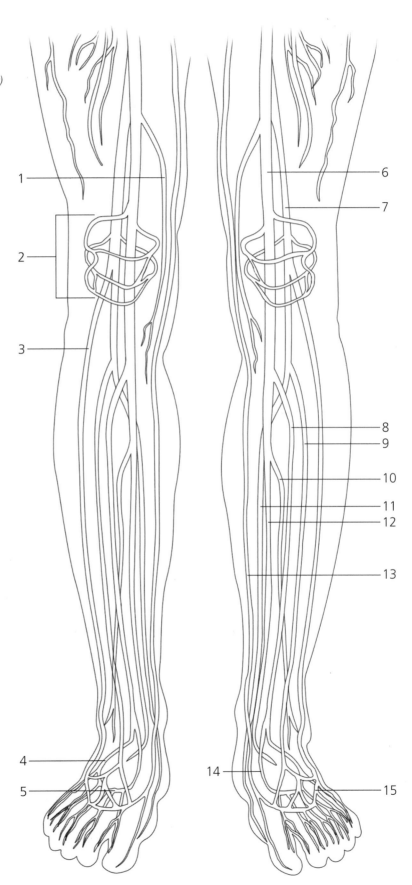

8.18

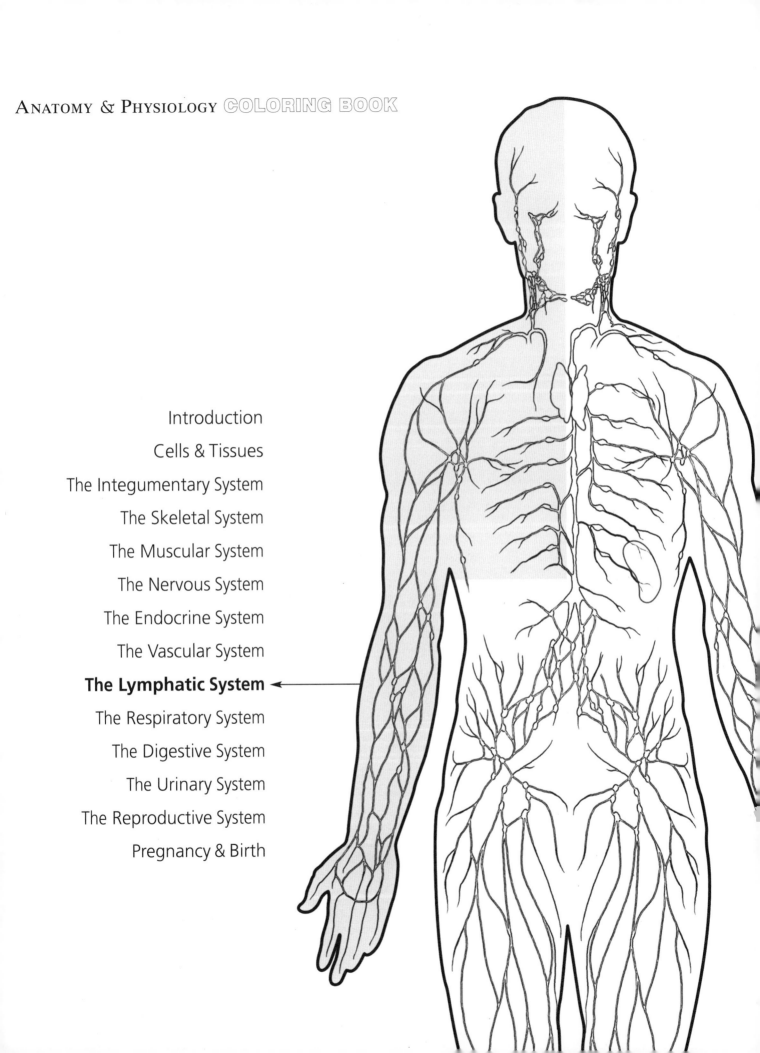

ANATOMY & PHYSIOLOGY COLORING BOOK

The LYMPHATIC System

System overview

The lymphatic system is an extensive network of vessels and nodes that forms a central part of the body's defenses against illness and injury. Foreign materials such as bacteria or dead cells are collected and transported through the lymph vessels, where they are filtered by the lymph nodes. The lymph vessels also drain excess fluid from the body's tissues, forming a fluid called **lymph**.

A – Right lymphatic drainage (*shaded*)
B – Left lymphatic drainage
○ 1. Right lymphatic duct
– 2. Axillary nodes
○ 3. Cisterna chyli
– 4. Lumbar nodes
– 5. Inguinal nodes
– 6. Popliteal nodes
○ 7. Left lymphatic duct
○ 8. Thoracic duct

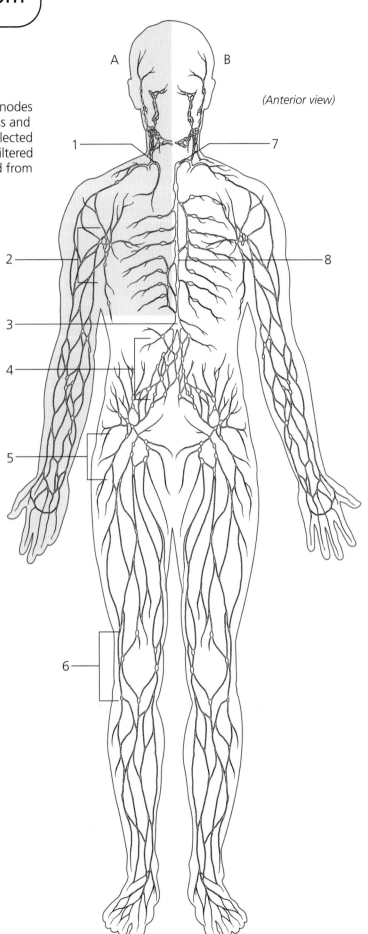

(Anterior view)

The LYMPHATIC System

Lymphatic drainage & lymphoid organs

(Anterior view)

○ 1. Popliteal nodes
○ 2. Tonsil
○ 3. Thymus
○ 4. Spleen
○ 5. Lymphatic vessel

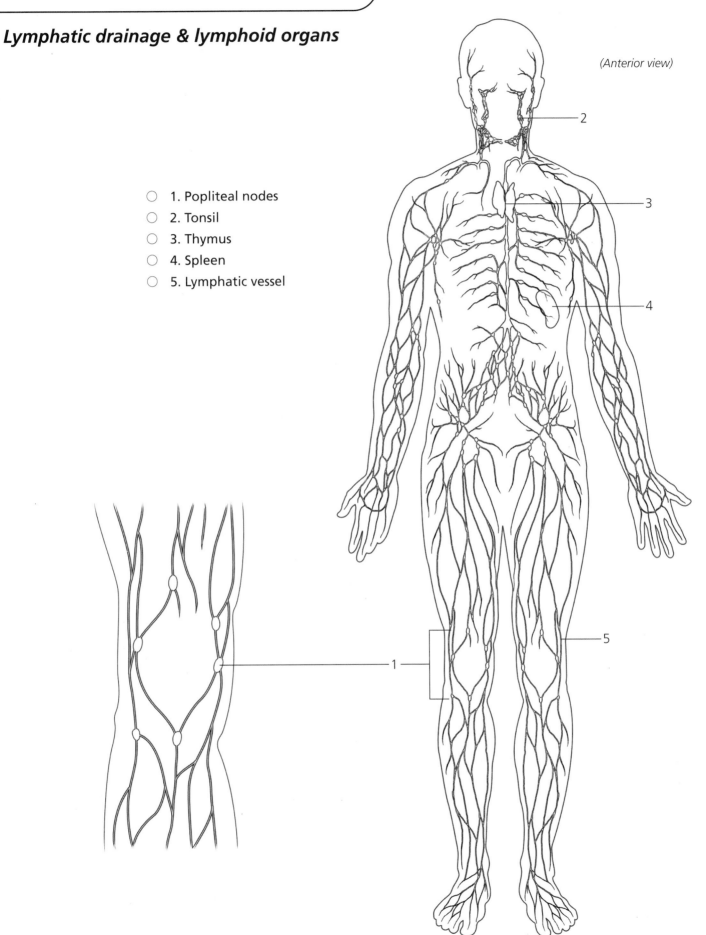

The LYMPHATIC System

Lymph & lymph vessels

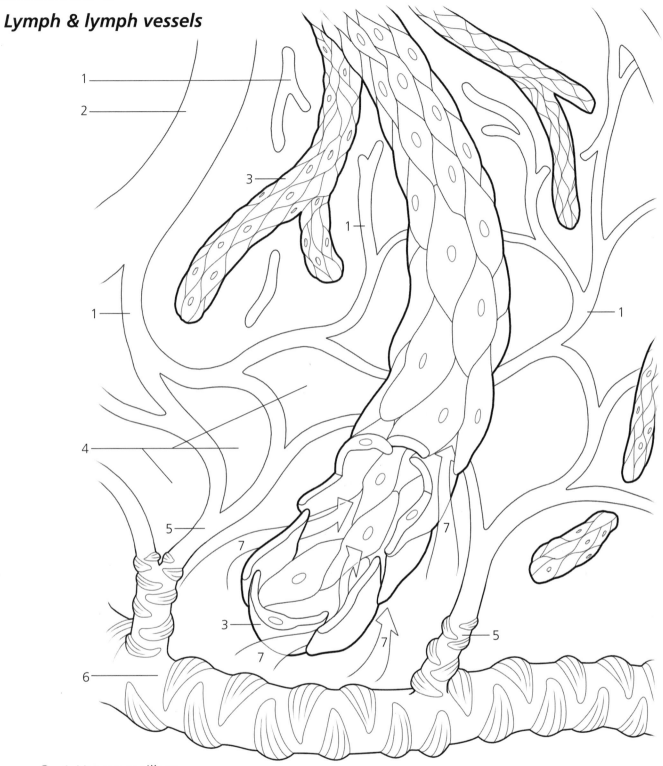

- ○ 1. Venous capillary
- ○ 2. Venule
- ○ 3. Lymphatic capillary
- − 4. Tissue cells and interstitial spaces
- ○ 5. Arterial capillary
- ○ 6. Arteriole
- ○ 7. Excess fluid

Lymph vessels begin as microscopic capillaries in intercellular spaces throughout the body and converge to form larger lymphatic vessels similar to veins. The lymph capillaries absorb excess fluid filtered from the blood to provide the tissues with oxygen and nutrients. Once inside the lymph vessels, this clear, watery **interstitial fluid** becomes known as **lymph**.

The LYMPHATIC System

Lymph node

(Sectional view)

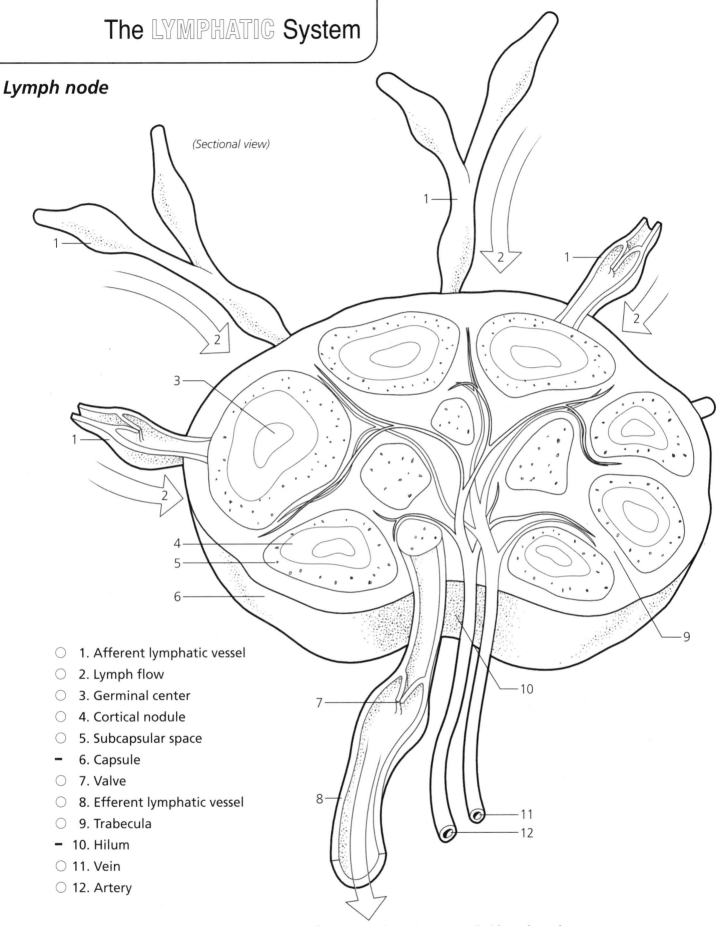

○ 1. Afferent lymphatic vessel
○ 2. Lymph flow
○ 3. Germinal center
○ 4. Cortical nodule
○ 5. Subcapsular space
− 6. Capsule
○ 7. Valve
○ 8. Efferent lymphatic vessel
○ 9. Trabecula
− 10. Hilum
○ 11. Vein
○ 12. Artery

The lymphatic vessels are lined with hundreds of tiny bean-shaped organs called **lymph nodes**. Although they are scattered throughout the body, large clusters of lymph nodes are concentrated near specific areas such as the **mammary glands** and **groin**. Lymph nodes act as a barrier to infection by scavenging bacteria and other foreign materials from the lymph collected from the organs and tissues before it is returned to the bloodstream.

The LYMPHATIC System

Lymph node

(Sectional view)

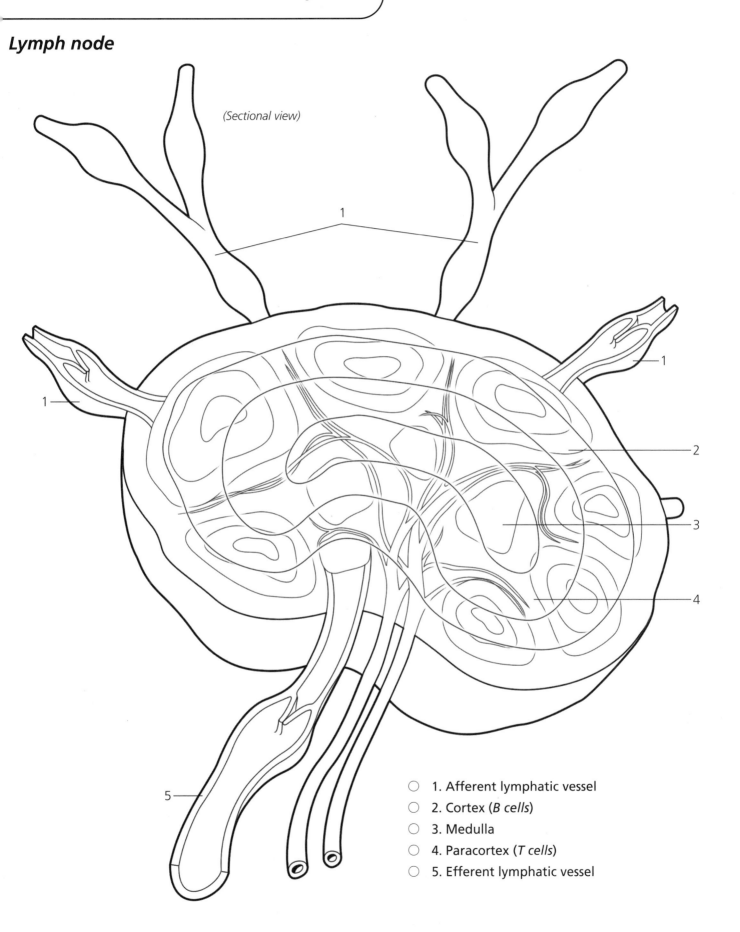

○ 1. Afferent lymphatic vessel
○ 2. Cortex (*B cells*)
○ 3. Medulla
○ 4. Paracortex (*T cells*)
○ 5. Efferent lymphatic vessel

The LYMPHATIC System

Secondary lymphatic organs

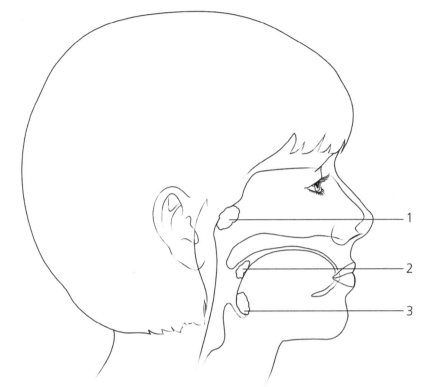

Tonsils

○ 1. Pharyngeal tonsil
○ 2. Palatine tonsil
○ 3. Lingual tonsil

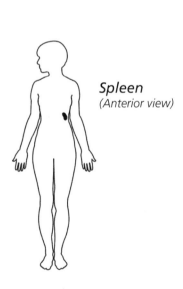

Spleen
(Anterior view)

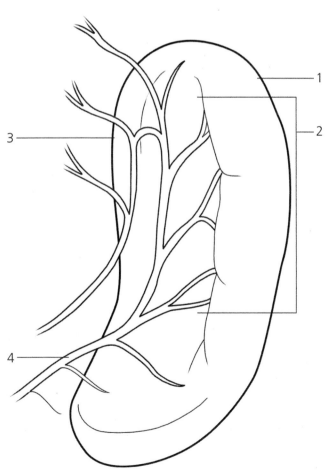

– 1. Diaphragmatic surface
– 2. Hilum
– 3. Visceral surface
○ 4. Spleen vein

The LYMPHATIC System

Regional lymphatic vessels

Lymph nodes of the breast
(Left breast – frontal view)

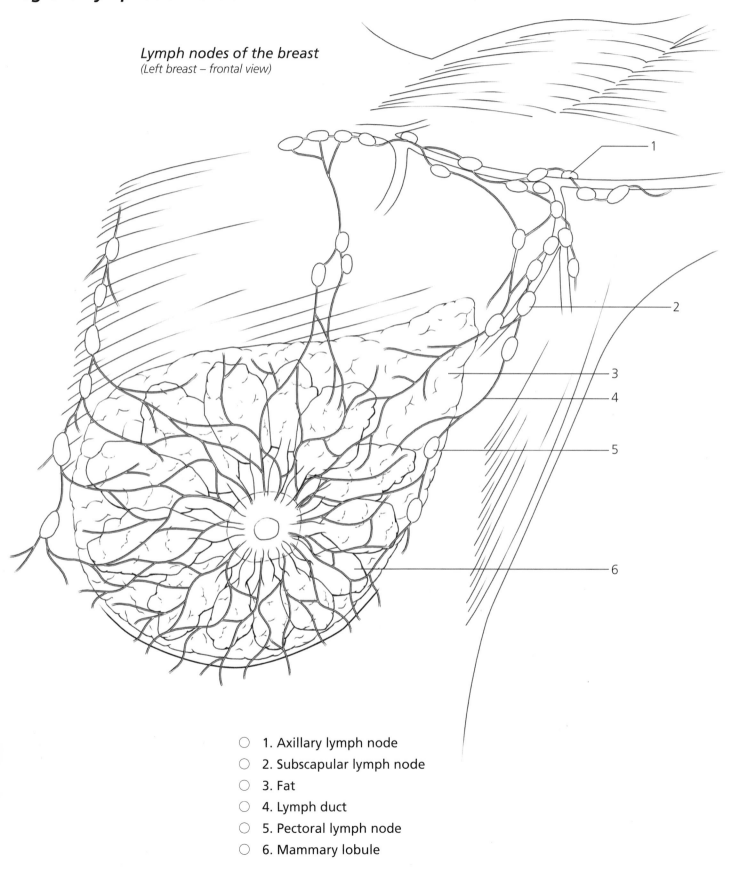

- ○ 1. Axillary lymph node
- ○ 2. Subscapular lymph node
- ○ 3. Fat
- ○ 4. Lymph duct
- ○ 5. Pectoral lymph node
- ○ 6. Mammary lobule

The LYMPHATIC System

Lymphocytes

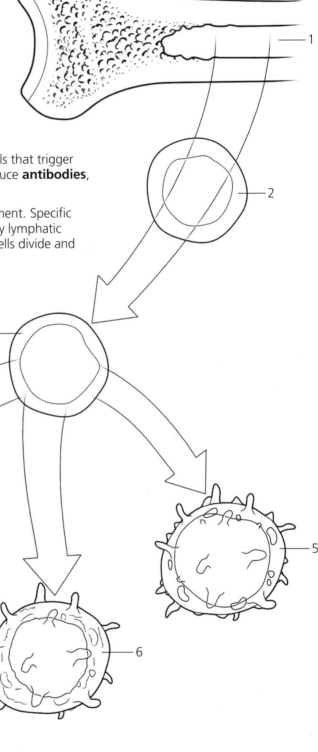

PHYSIOLOGY:
Lymphocyte formation

The lymphatic system contains millions of **lymphocytes**, cells that trigger immune responses, target and destroy pathogens, and produce **antibodies**, proteins that inactivate specific antigens.

All lymphocytes originate as stem cells during fetal development. Specific lymphocyte growth and production take place in the primary lymphatic organs (bone marrow and thymus gland), where the stem cells divide and mature into B, T and NK cells.

○ 1. Red bone marrow

○ 2. Stem cell

○ 3. Lymphoid progenitor cell

○ 4. Thymus

○ 5. NK cell

○ 6. B cell

○ 7. T cell

ANATOMY & PHYSIOLOGY COLORING BOOK

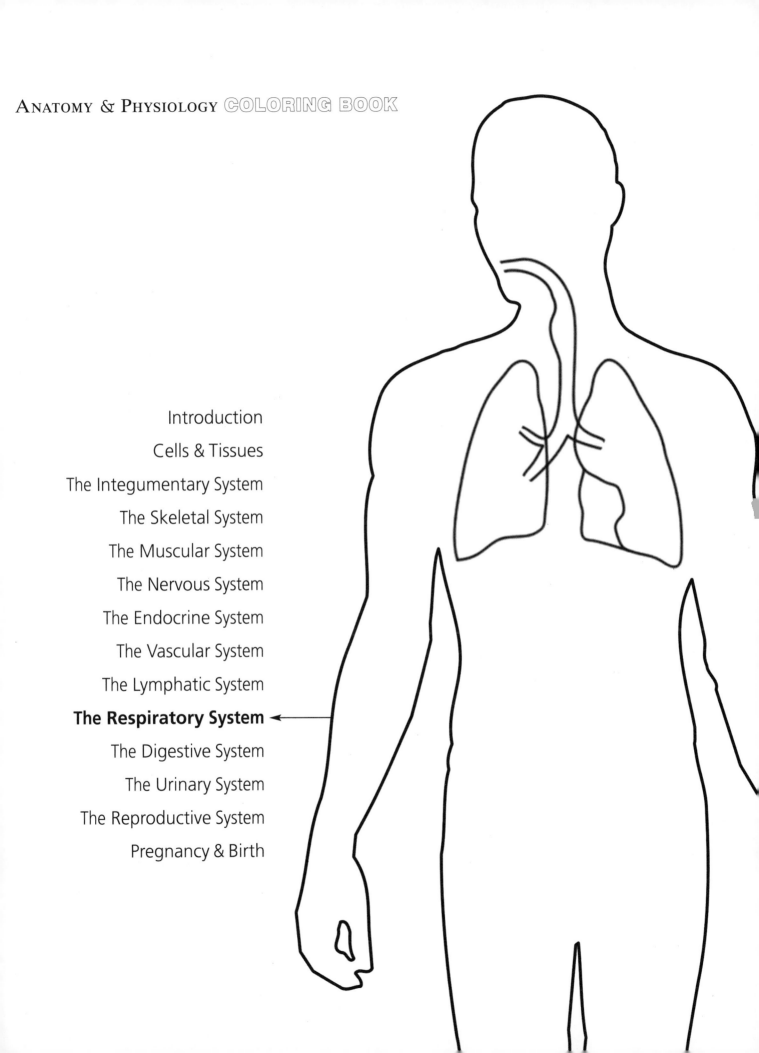

System overview

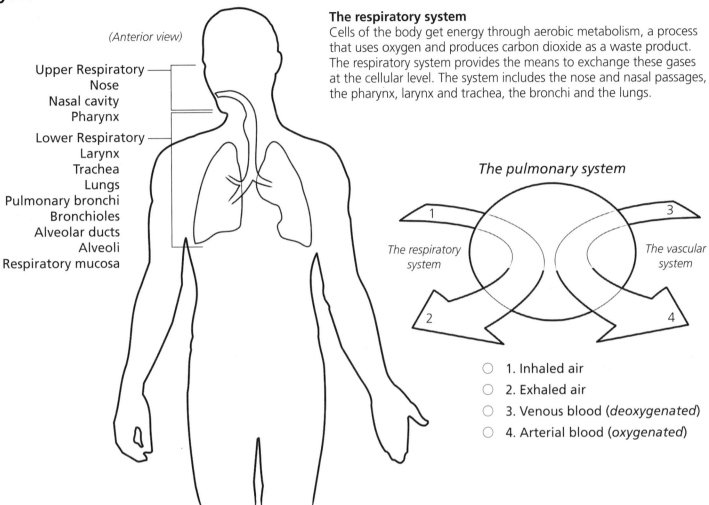

(Anterior view)

Upper Respiratory
Nose
Nasal cavity
Pharynx

Lower Respiratory
Larynx
Trachea
Lungs
Pulmonary bronchi
Bronchioles
Alveolar ducts
Alveoli
Respiratory mucosa

The respiratory system
Cells of the body get energy through aerobic metabolism, a process that uses oxygen and produces carbon dioxide as a waste product. The respiratory system provides the means to exchange these gases at the cellular level. The system includes the nose and nasal passages, the pharynx, larynx and trachea, the bronchi and the lungs.

The pulmonary system

The respiratory system   *The vascular system*

○ 1. Inhaled air
○ 2. Exhaled air
○ 3. Venous blood (*deoxygenated*)
○ 4. Arterial blood (*oxygenated*)

Pulmonary circulation
The right ventricle of the heart pumps blood to the pulmonary artery, which branches into the left and right sides of the lungs. The pulmonary arteries divide and form pulmonary capillaries surrounding the alveoli. The capillaries then join together to form venules and veins, providing a pathway to return oxygenated blood to the left atrium of the heart.

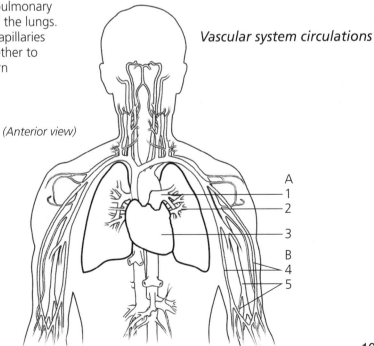

Vascular system circulations

(Anterior view)

A – Pulmonary circulation
    ○ 1. Pulmonary arteries
    ○ 2. Pulmonary veins
○ 3. Cardiac circulation
B – Systemic circulation
    ○ 4. Veins
    ○ 5. Arteries

The RESPIRATORY System

PHYSIOLOGY:
Breathing: Upper respiratory tract

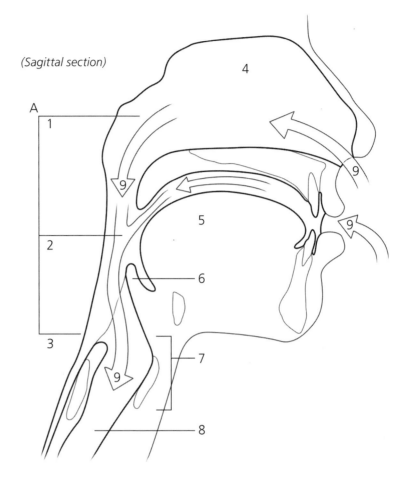

(Sagittal section)

A – Pharynx
- — 1. Nasopharynx
- — 2. Oropharynx
- — 3. Laryngopharynx
- ○ 4. Nasal passages
- ○ 5. Tongue
- ○ 6. Epiglottis
- — 7. Larynx
- ○ 8. Trachea
- ○ 9. Air

Pulmonary function test
One second forced expiratory volume (FEV_1)

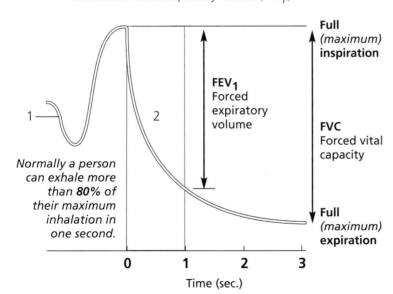

Full (maximum) inspiration

FEV_1 Forced expiratory volume

FVC Forced vital capacity

Full (maximum) expiration

*Normally a person can exhale more than **80%** of their maximum inhalation in one second.*

Time (sec.)

Through breathing, the respiratory system provides needed oxygen and expels carbon dioxide. A complete breath includes taking air into the lungs (**inspiration**) and then expelling it (**expiration**).

The upper respiratory system consists of the nose, nasal passages, paranasal sinuses and pharynx. The paranasal sinuses are hollow cavities within the bones of the face behind the eyes and around the nose. There are four pairs of sinuses: frontal, maxillary, ethmoid and sphenoid. They are joined by a continuous mucous membrane that produces **mucus**, a slippery secretion that moistens the nasal passages and traps dirt particles from incoming air.

- ○ 1. Volume of air in lung
- ○ 2. One second exhale

The RESPIRATORY System

Paranasal sinuses

○ 1. Frontal sinus
○ 2. Nasal septum
○ 3. Nasal cavity
○ 4. Maxillary sinus
○ 5. Sphenoid sinus
○ 6. Ethmoid cells
○ 7. Frontal sinus
– 8. Opening of right
      maxillary sinus
○ 9. Nasal cavity

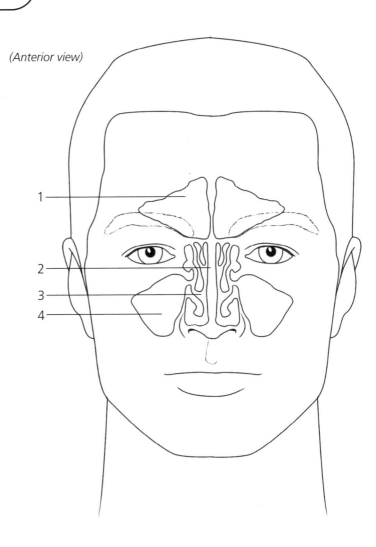

(Sagittal section)

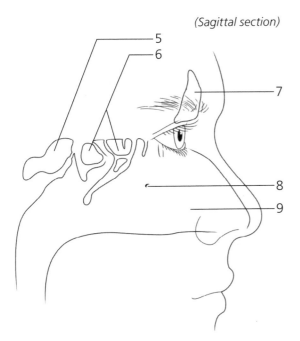

Respiratory epithelium
(Diagrammatic view)

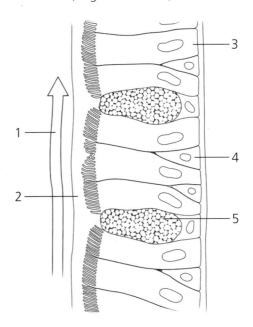

○ 1. Mucus movement
      toward the pharynx
○ 2. Mucous layer
○ 3. Ciliated columnar
      epithelial cell
○ 4. Stem cell
○ 5. Mucous cell

The RESPIRATORY System

Larynx

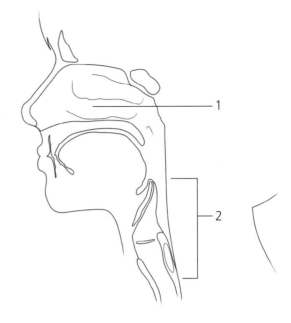

(Sagittal section)

○ 1. Nasal passages
– 2. Larynx
○ 3. Epiglottis
○ 4. Hyoid bone
○ 5. Thyroid cartilage
○ 6. Arytenoid cartilage
○ 7. Cricoid cartilage
○ 8. Hyoepiglottic ligament

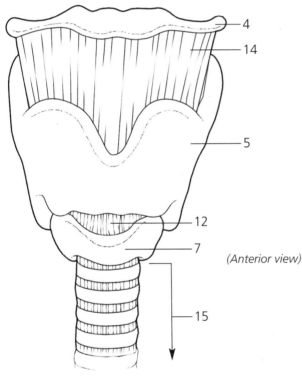

(Anterior view)

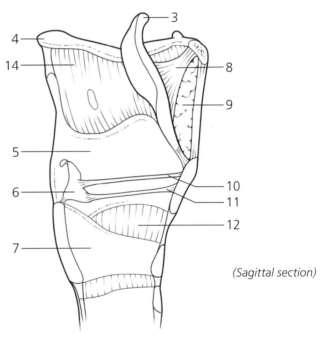

(Sagittal section)

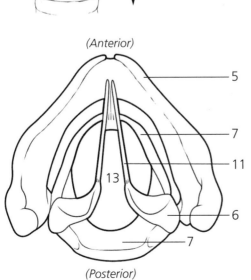

(Anterior)

(Posterior)

Coloring guide suggestion
When coloring, use same color to indicate similar parts

○ 9. Pre-epiglottic fat body
○ 10. Vestibular ligament
○ 11. Vocal ligament
○ 12. Cricothyroid ligament
– 13. Glottis
○ 14. Thyrohyoid membrane
○ 15. Trachea

The RESPIRATORY System

Chest wall

Left lung
(Partial coronal section)

1. Superior lobe
2. Inferior lobe
3. Intercostal muscle
4. Diaphragm
5. External intercostal muscle
6. Internal intercostal muscle
7. Innermost intercostal muscle

8. Parietal pleura
9. Pleural cavity
10. Visceral pleura
11. Rib
12. Lung
13. Intercostal vein, artery and nerve

Layers of the chest wall

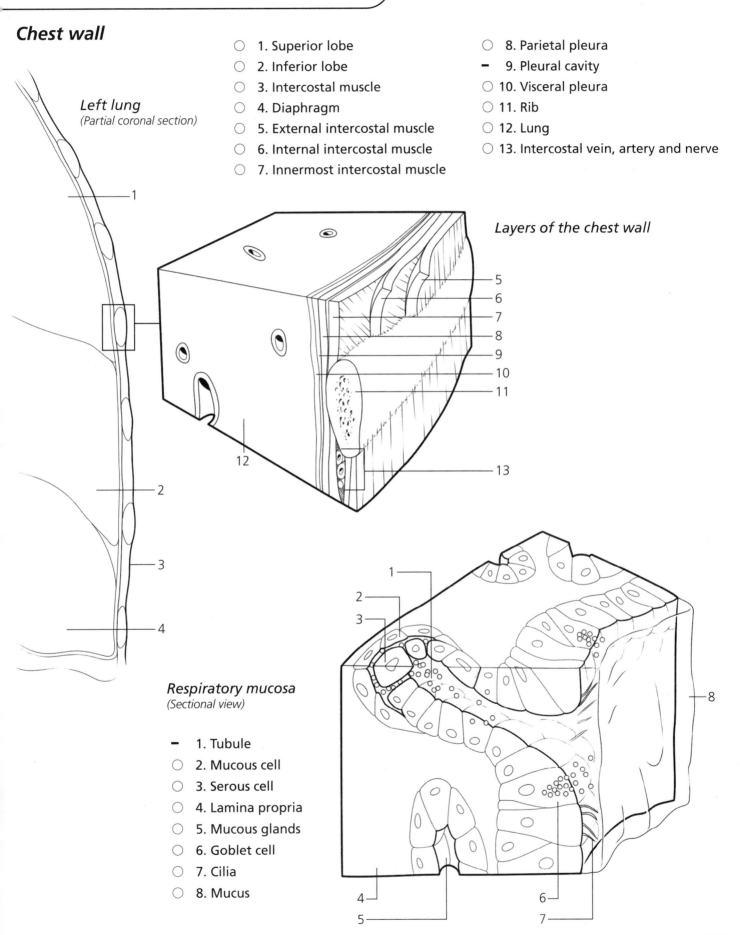

Respiratory mucosa
(Sectional view)

1. Tubule
2. Mucous cell
3. Serous cell
4. Lamina propria
5. Mucous glands
6. Goblet cell
7. Cilia
8. Mucus

Bronchopulmonary segments

A – Superior lobe (*right lung*)
- ○ 1. Apical
- ○ 2. Posterior
- ○ 3. Anterior

B – Middle lobe (*right lung*)
- ○ 4. Medial
- ○ 5. Lateral

C – Inferior lobe (*right lung*)
- ○ 6. Anterior basal
- ○ 7. Lateral basal
- ○ 8. Posterior basal
- ○ 9. Medial basal

D – Superior lobe (*left lung*)
- ○ 10. Apical
- ○ 11. Anterior
- ○ 12. Superior lingular
- ○ 13. Inferior lingular

E – Inferior lobe (*left lung*)
- ○ 14. Medial basal
- ○ 15. Lateral basal
- ○ 16. Posterior basal

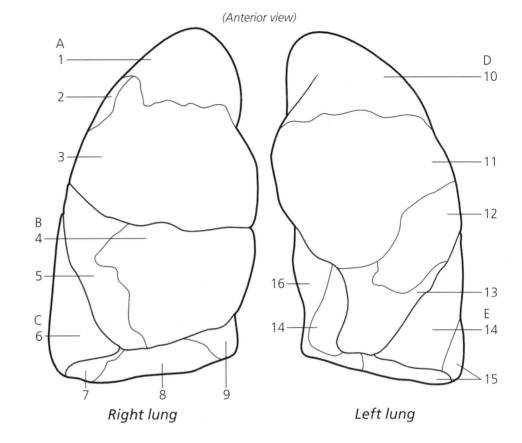

(Anterior view)

Right lung   *Left lung*

A – Superior lobe (*left lung*)
- ○ 1. Apicoposterior
- ○ 2. Anterior
- ○ 3. Superior lingular

B – Inferior lobe (*left lung*)
- ○ 4. Superior
- ○ 5. Lateral basal
- ○ 6. Posterior basal

C – Superior lobe (*right lung*)
- ○ 7. Apicoposterior
- ○ 8. Posterior
- ○ 9. Anterior

D – Middle lobe (*right lung*)
- ○ 10. Lateral

E – Inferior lobe (*right lung*)
- ○ 11. Superior
- ○ 12. Anterior basal
- ○ 13. Lateral basal
- ○ 14. Posterior basal

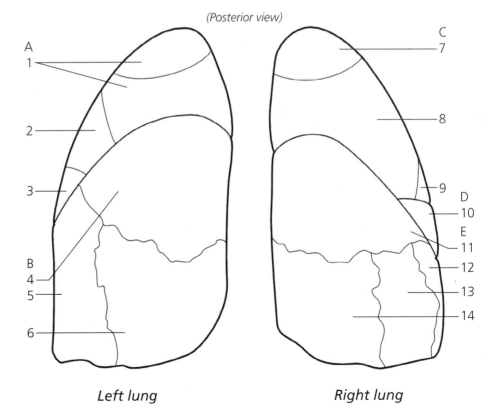

(Posterior view)

Left lung   *Right lung*

10.6

The RESPIRATORY System

Bronchi

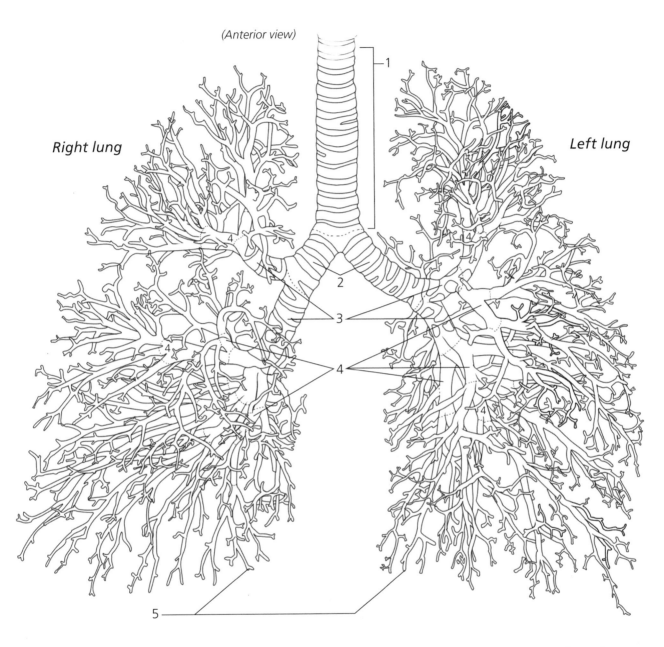

(Anterior view)

Right lung

Left lung

1

2

3

4

4

5

There are three secondary bronchi in the
right lung, but only two in the left lung.

○ 1. Tracheal
○ 2. Trachea bronchus
○ 3. Secondary bronchus

○ 4. Tertiary bronchus
○ 5. Terminal bronchioles

Coloring guide suggestion
*When coloring the bronchus
extend color to dotted line*
- - - - - - - - - - -

Bronchioles

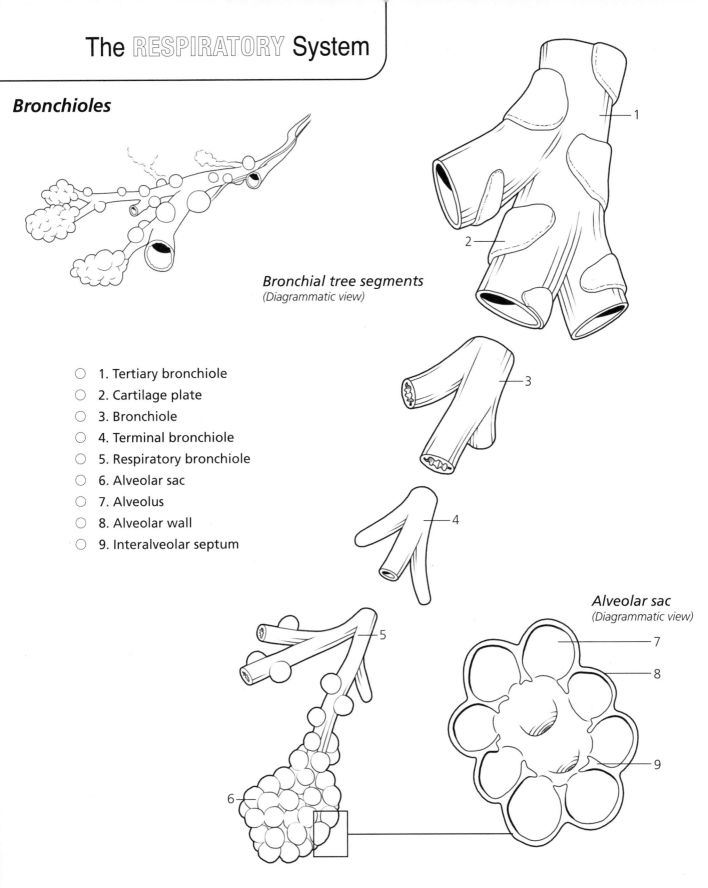

Bronchial tree segments
(Diagrammatic view)

○ 1. Tertiary bronchiole
○ 2. Cartilage plate
○ 3. Bronchiole
○ 4. Terminal bronchiole
○ 5. Respiratory bronchiole
○ 6. Alveolar sac
○ 7. Alveolus
○ 8. Alveolar wall
○ 9. Interalveolar septum

Alveolar sac
(Diagrammatic view)

Elastic recoil

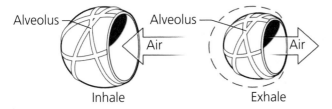

Alveolus — Alveolus
Air   Air
Inhale   Exhale

The **alveoli** are covered by elastic fibers.
After the alveoli expand during inhalation,
the recoil of these fibers causes the alveoli
to contract, helping the process of exhalation.

The RESPIRATORY System

PHYSIOLOGY:
Respiration

During inhalation, the diaphragm moves down as it contracts, and the intercostal muscles lift as they pull the ribs outward. These actions increase the volume of the chest cavity. A partial vacuum is created by the additional space, and air is drawn in to equalize the pressure.

- ○ 1. Lung
- ○ 2. Sternum
- − 3. External intercostal muscle
- − 4. Ribs
- ○ 5. Diaphragm
- ○ 6. Nitrogen
- ○ 7. Oxygen
- − 8. Water vapor
- − 9. Carbon dioxide

During exhalation, the intercostal and diaphragm muscles relax, contracting the chest cavity. Air is pushed out of the lungs as they passively recoil.

- ○ 1. Lung
- ○ 2. Sternum
- − 3. External intercostal muscle
- − 4. Ribs
- ○ 5. Diaphragm
- ○ 6. Nitrogen
- ○ 7. Oxygen
- ○ 8. Water vapor
- ○ 9. Carbon dioxide

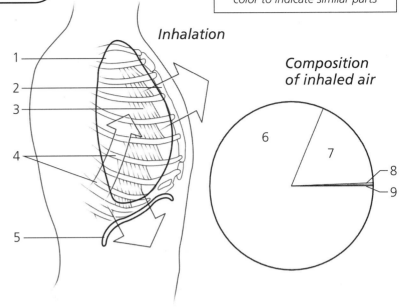

Inhalation

Composition of inhaled air

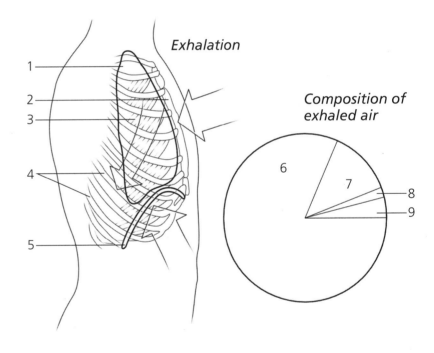

Exhalation

Composition of exhaled air

PHYSIOLOGY:
Lung volumes

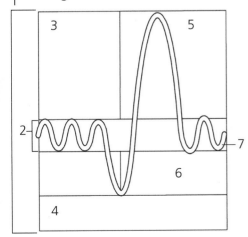

During normal respiration, the amount of air breathed in and out is called **tidal volume**. The additional amount of air that can be forcibly inhaled (past a normal inhalation) is the **inspiratory reserve volume**. The additional amount of air that can be forcibly exhaled (past a normal exhalation) is the **expiratory reserve volume**. Together the inspiratory reserve volume and the expiratory reserve volume make up the **vital capacity**. Exhaling all the air in our lungs would create a vacuum, so some air remains in the lungs. This air is called **residual volume**. Adding the residual volume to the vital capacity gives us the **total lung capacity** (almost six liters of air).

- − 1. Total lung capacity
- ○ 2. Tidal volume
- ○ 3. Vital capacity
- ○ 4. Residual volume
- ○ 5. Inspiratory reserve volume
- ○ 6. Expiratory reserve volume
- ○ 7. Breathing

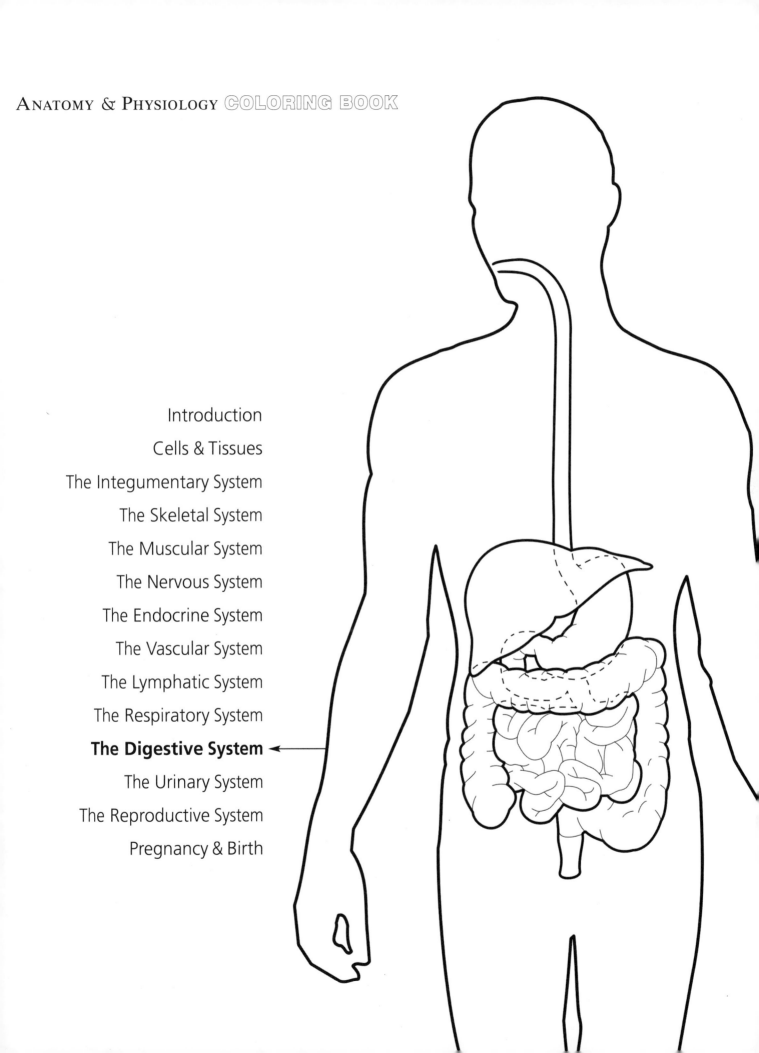

ANATOMY & PHYSIOLOGY COLORING BOOK

The DIGESTIVE System

System overview

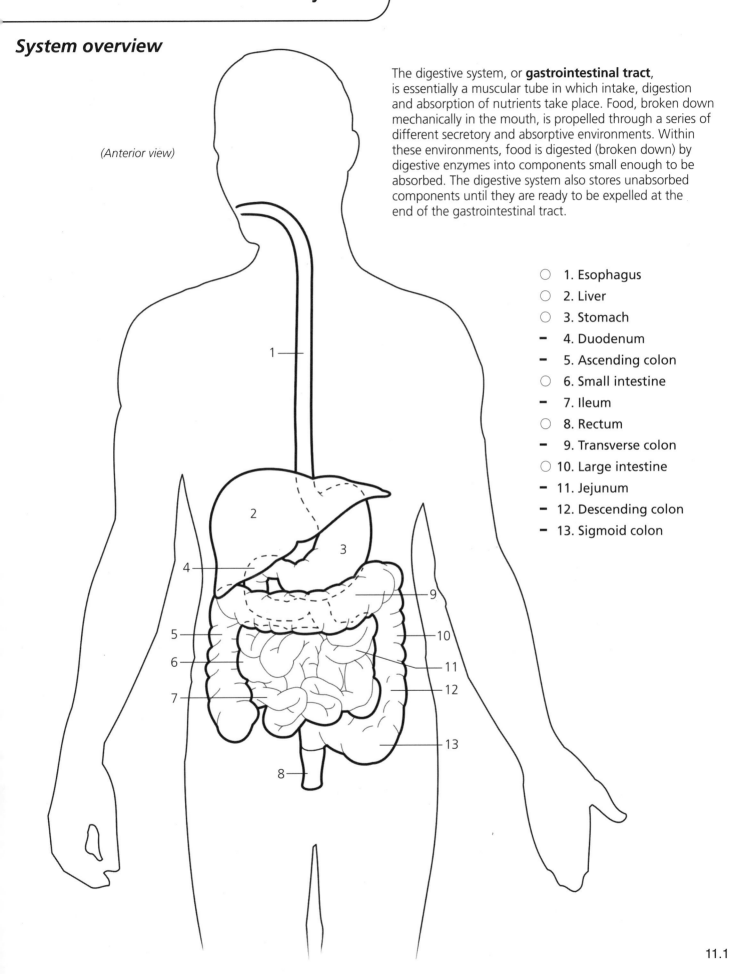

(Anterior view)

The digestive system, or **gastrointestinal tract**, is essentially a muscular tube in which intake, digestion and absorption of nutrients take place. Food, broken down mechanically in the mouth, is propelled through a series of different secretory and absorptive environments. Within these environments, food is digested (broken down) by digestive enzymes into components small enough to be absorbed. The digestive system also stores unabsorbed components until they are ready to be expelled at the end of the gastrointestinal tract.

○ 1. Esophagus
○ 2. Liver
○ 3. Stomach
– 4. Duodenum
– 5. Ascending colon
○ 6. Small intestine
– 7. Ileum
○ 8. Rectum
– 9. Transverse colon
○ 10. Large intestine
– 11. Jejunum
– 12. Descending colon
– 13. Sigmoid colon

The DIGESTIVE System

The digestive system

PHYSIOLOGY:
The digestive process

Once in the stomach, food is churned and mixed with hydrochloric acid and enzymes to begin the digestion of proteins. The stomach also functions to store chyme, or partially digested food, for processing later by the small intestine. After leaving the stomach, chyme moves into the duodenum, the first part of the small intestine, where it is mixed with bile produced by the liver and pancreatic juice produced by the pancreas. Excess bile is stored in the gallbladder. As undigested material moves through the large intestine, water and electrolytes are absorbed (**dehydration**). The remaining waste is stored, formed and expelled (**elimination**).

A – Ingestion
B – Digestion
C – Digestion and absorption
D – Absorption and dehydration
E – Elimination
○ 1. Esophagus
○ 2. Stomach
○ 3. Small intestine
○ 4. Large intestine
○ 5. Rectum

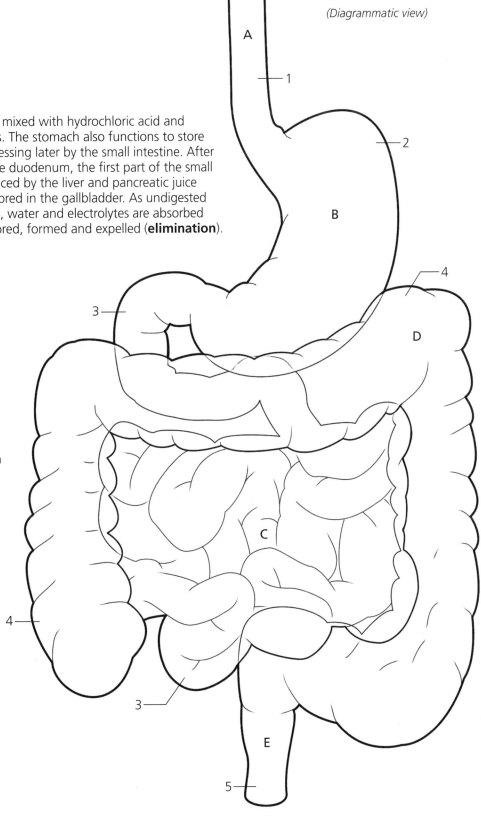

(Diagrammatic view)

The digestive system

(Diagrammatic view)

PHYSIOLOGY:
Swallowing

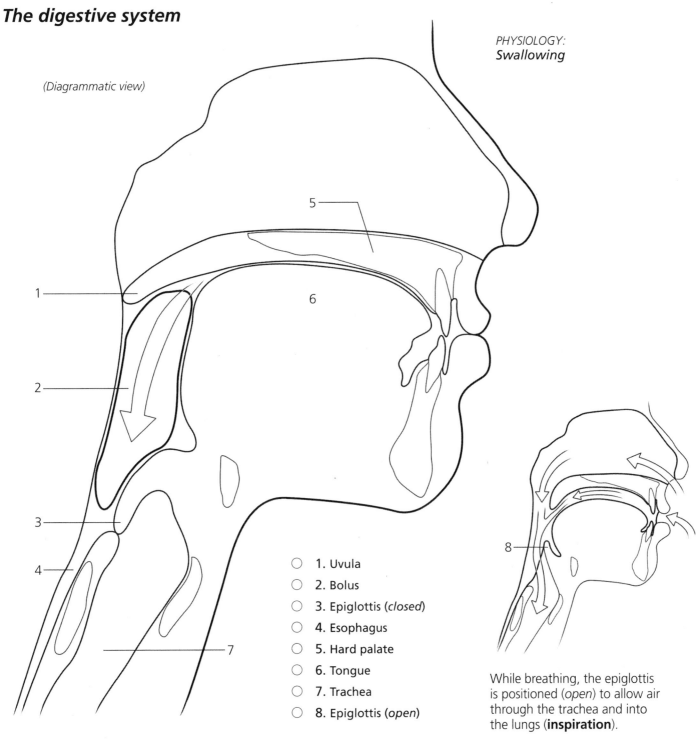

○ 1. Uvula
○ 2. Bolus
○ 3. Epiglottis (*closed*)
○ 4. Esophagus
○ 5. Hard palate
○ 6. Tongue
○ 7. Trachea
○ 8. Epiglottis (*open*)

While breathing, the epiglottis is positioned (*open*) to allow air through the trachea and into the lungs (**inspiration**).

Without the ability of the epiglottis to close during swallowing, food, saliva or foreign objects would enter the airways (**aspiration**).

Chewing, the mechanical action involving the teeth and tongue, begins the breakdown of solid food. This greatly increases food's surface area and mixes the food with saliva, a secretion of the salivary glands. Saliva moistens the food and begins the digestion of starch. The mixture of food and saliva is called a bolus. As the bolus leaves the pharynx, the epiglottis, a flap-like valve, and the vocal cords close, blocking the trachea. Peristaltic action moves the bolus through the esophagus to the stomach.

The digestive system

(Diagrammatic view)

PHYSIOLOGY:
Peristaltic action

Material is moved through the digestive system by a series of muscle contractions called peristalsis. The muscle behind the material contracts, while the muscle ahead relaxes, moving the material into the next section.

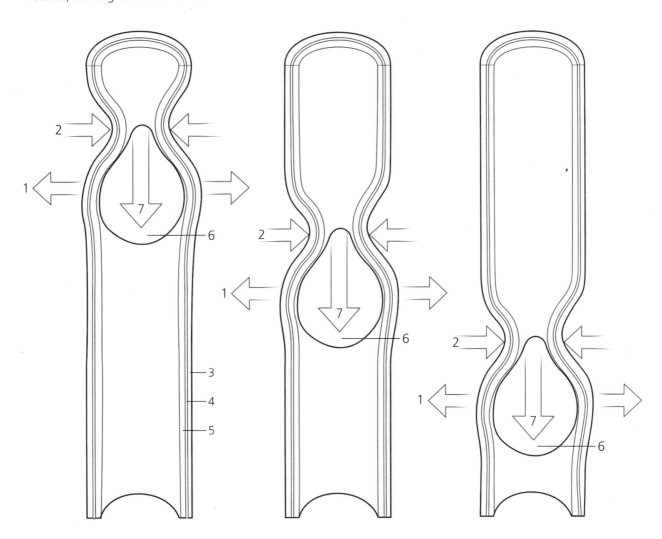

○ 1. Relax

○ 2. Contract

○ 3. Serosa (*adventitia*)

○ 4. Muscularis externa

○ 5. Mucosa and submucosa

○ 6. Material

○ 7. Direction of movement

The DIGESTIVE System

The stomach

(Frontal view – section removed for clarity)

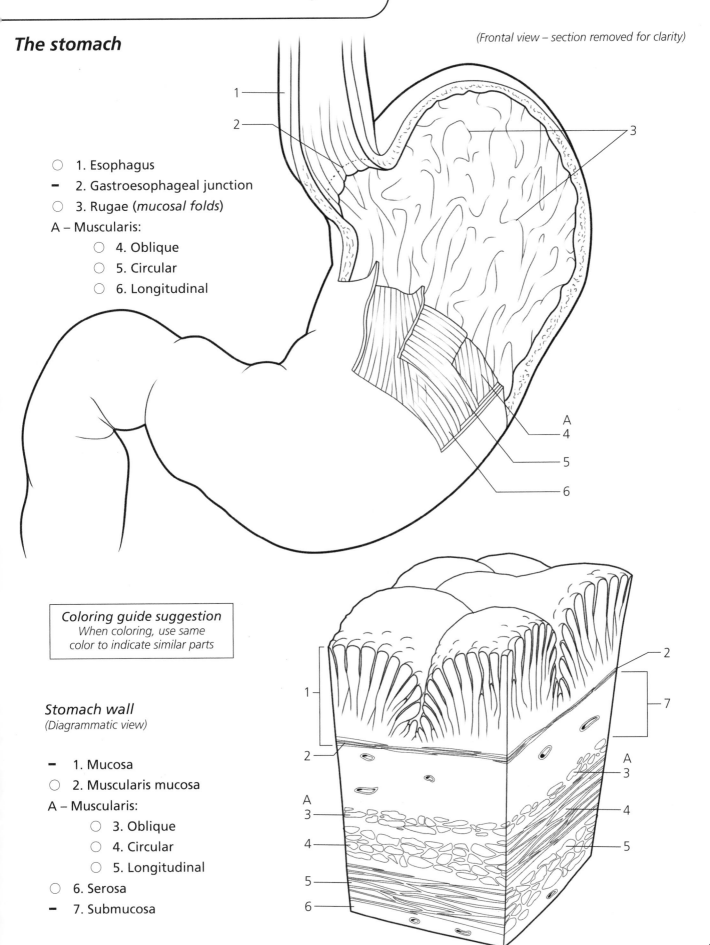

○ 1. Esophagus
− 2. Gastroesophageal junction
○ 3. Rugae (*mucosal folds*)
A – Muscularis:
    ○ 4. Oblique
    ○ 5. Circular
    ○ 6. Longitudinal

Coloring guide suggestion
*When coloring, use same
color to indicate similar parts*

Stomach wall
(Diagrammatic view)

− 1. Mucosa
○ 2. Muscularis mucosa
A – Muscularis:
    ○ 3. Oblique
    ○ 4. Circular
    ○ 5. Longitudinal
○ 6. Serosa
− 7. Submucosa

11.5

The DIGESTIVE System

Gastric gland

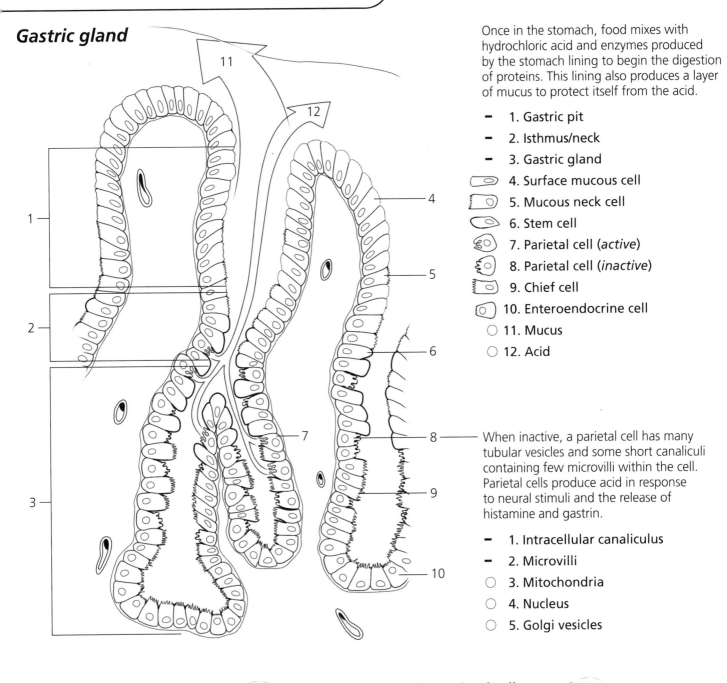

Once in the stomach, food mixes with hydrochloric acid and enzymes produced by the stomach lining to begin the digestion of proteins. This lining also produces a layer of mucus to protect itself from the acid.

- 1. Gastric pit
- 2. Isthmus/neck
- 3. Gastric gland
- 4. Surface mucous cell
- 5. Mucous neck cell
- 6. Stem cell
- 7. Parietal cell (*active*)
- 8. Parietal cell (*inactive*)
- 9. Chief cell
- 10. Enteroendocrine cell
- 11. Mucus
- 12. Acid

When inactive, a parietal cell has many tubular vesicles and some short canaliculi containing few microvilli within the cell. Parietal cells produce acid in response to neural stimuli and the release of histamine and gastrin.

- 1. Intracellular canaliculus
- 2. Microvilli
- 3. Mitochondria
- 4. Nucleus
- 5. Golgi vesicles

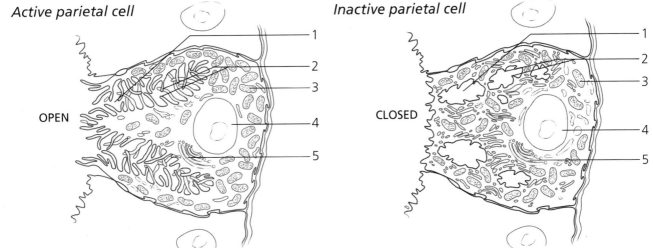

Active parietal cell

OPEN

Inactive parietal cell

CLOSED

The DIGESTIVE System

The small intestine

(Frontal view – section removed for clarity)

- — 1. Pyloric sphincter
- ○ 2. Duodenum
- ○ 3. Ileum
- ○ 4. Ileocecal valve
  (opening *to large intestine*)
- ○ 5. Jejunum
- — 6. Plicae circulares (*ridges*)
- ○ 7. Mesentery

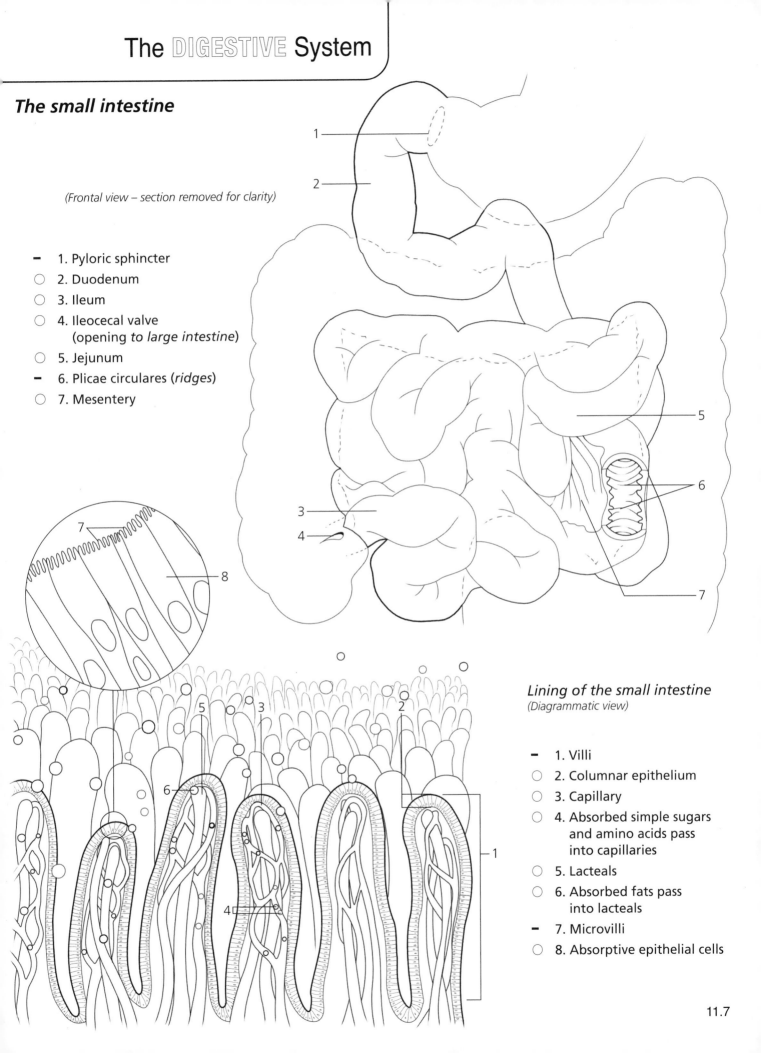

Lining of the small intestine
(*Diagrammatic view*)

- — 1. Villi
- ○ 2. Columnar epithelium
- ○ 3. Capillary
- ○ 4. Absorbed simple sugars
  and amino acids pass
  into capillaries
- ○ 5. Lacteals
- ○ 6. Absorbed fats pass
  into lacteals
- — 7. Microvilli
- ○ 8. Absorptive epithelial cells

The DIGESTIVE System

The large intestine

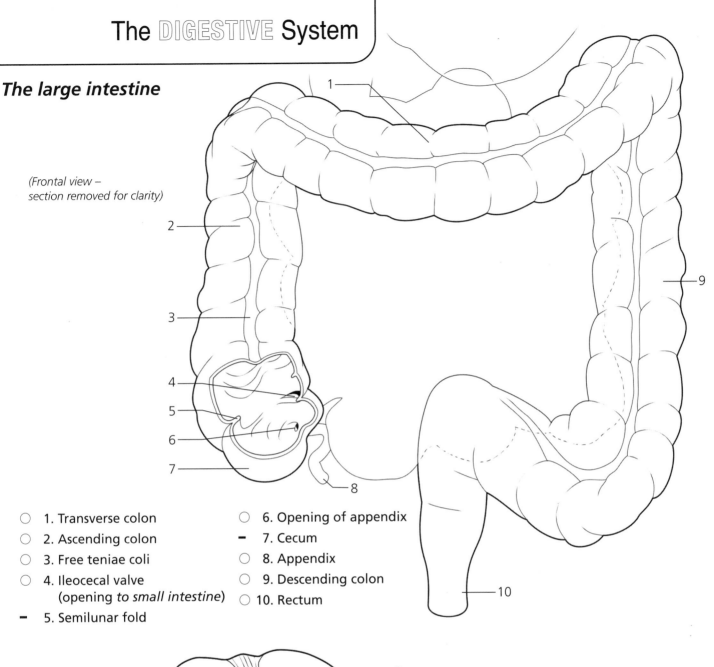

(Frontal view – section removed for clarity)

○ 1. Transverse colon
○ 2. Ascending colon
○ 3. Free teniae coli
○ 4. Ileocecal valve
   (opening *to small intestine*)
– 5. Semilunar fold

○ 6. Opening of appendix
– 7. Cecum
○ 8. Appendix
○ 9. Descending colon
○ 10. Rectum

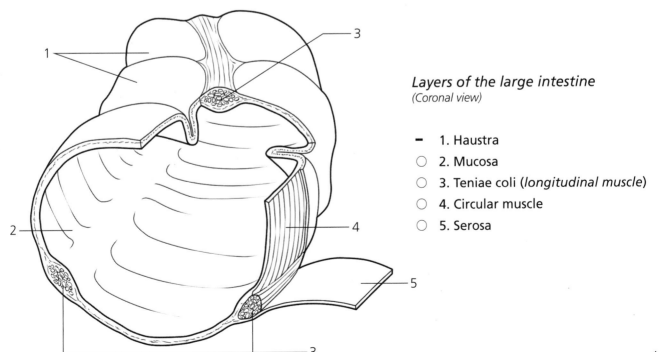

Layers of the large intestine
(Coronal view)

– 1. Haustra
○ 2. Mucosa
○ 3. Teniae coli (*longitudinal muscle*)
○ 4. Circular muscle
○ 5. Serosa

11.8

The DIGESTIVE System

Types of movement

PHYSIOLOGY:
Colonic movement

- 1. Transverse colon
- ○ 2. Segmentation
- 3. Ascending colon
- ○ 4. Peristaltic action
- 5. Descending colon
- ○ 6. Mass movement
- 7. Rectum

Movement through the large intestine is accomplished through the contractions of the longitudinal and circular musculature. Types of movement include peristaltic action, segmentation and mass movement. Movement of feces through the large intestine is slower than through the small intestine, allowing for reabsorption of water.

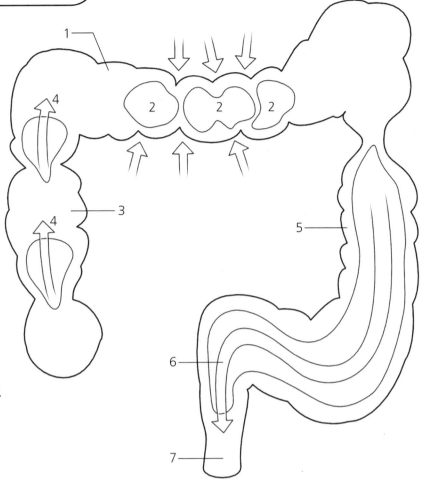

PHYSIOLOGY:
Segmentation

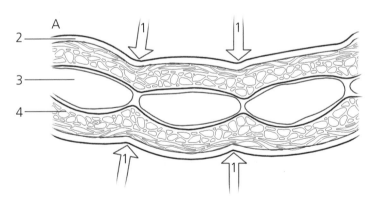

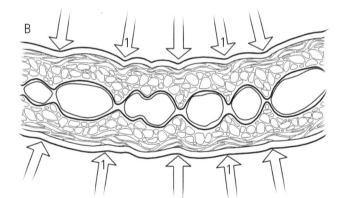

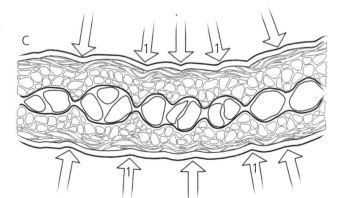

A – Muscle contractions begin to break up the material

B – Continuing muscle contractions produce further mixing

C – The waste material has been mixed, but not moved

- ○ 1. Muscle contractions
- ○ 2. Longitudinal muscles
- ○ 3. Ingested material
- ○ 4. Circular muscles

At regular intervals, ring-like contractions churn and mix the waste material, but do not move the material along. This process is called **segmentation**.

11.9

The liver

(Anterior view)

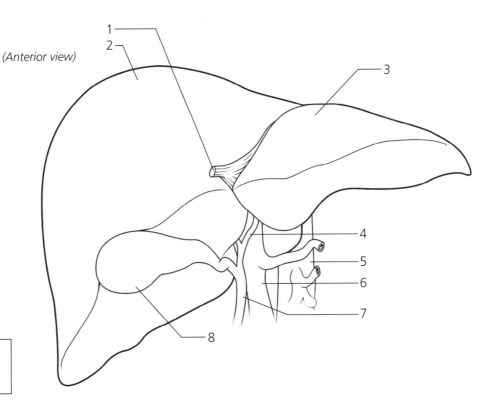

- — 1. Falciform ligament (*cut*)
- ○ 2. Right lobe
- ○ 3. Left lobe
- ○ 4. Common hepatic duct
- ○ 5. Aorta
- ○ 6. Portal vein
- ○ 7. Common bile duct
- ○ 8. Gallbladder

Coloring guide suggestion
When coloring, use same color to indicate similar parts

(Visceral surface)

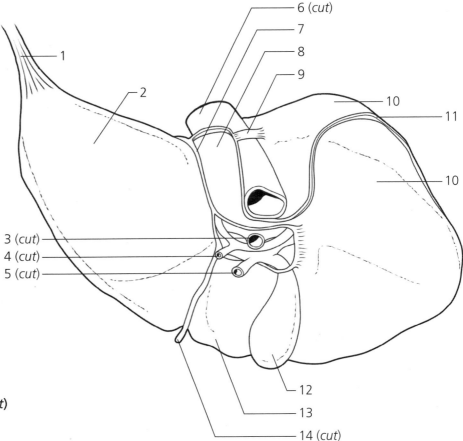

- — 1. Fibrous appendix of the liver (*triangular ligament*)
- ○ 2. Left lobe
- ○ 3. Hepatic artery (*cut*)
- ○ 4. Portal vein (*cut*)
- ○ 5. Bile duct (*cut*)
- ○ 6. Inferior vena cava (*cut*)
- — 7. Ligamentum venosum
- ○ 8. Caudate lobe
- — 9. Ligament of the inferior vena cava
- ○ 10. Right lobe
- — 11. Coronary ligament of the liver
- ○ 12. Gallbladder
- ○ 13. Quadrate lobe
- — 14. Round ligament of the liver (*cut*)

Liver lobules

(Frontal view – sections removed for clarity)

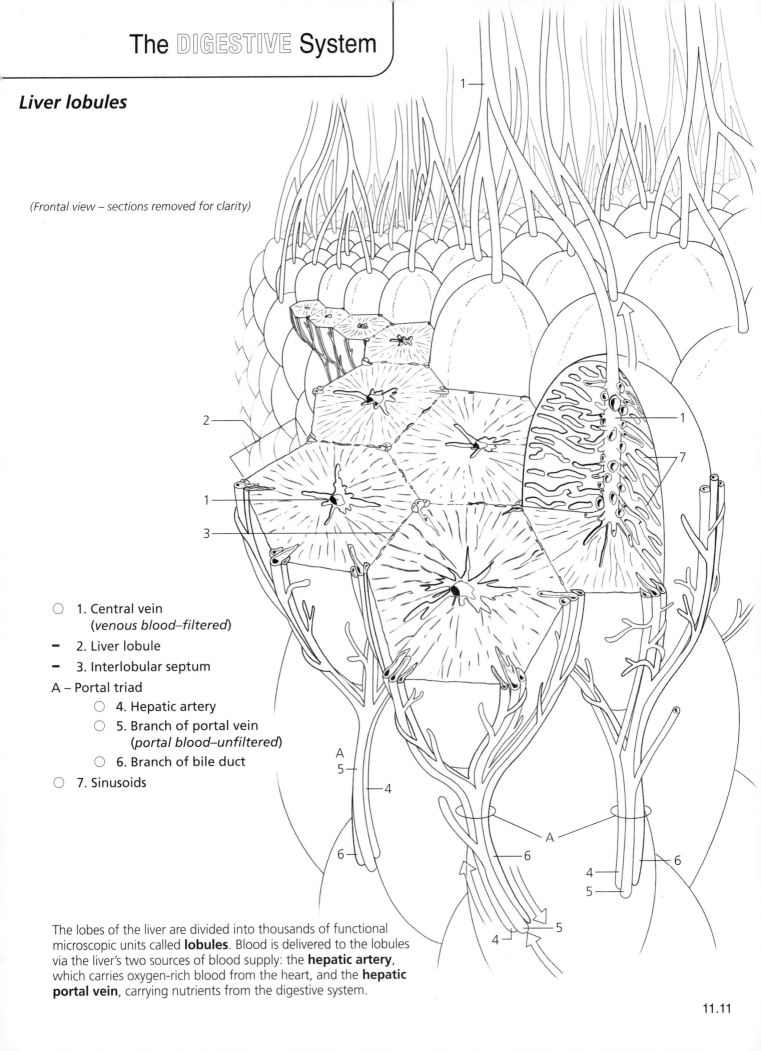

○ 1. Central vein
   (*venous blood–filtered*)

— 2. Liver lobule

— 3. Interlobular septum

A – Portal triad

   ○ 4. Hepatic artery

   ○ 5. Branch of portal vein
      (*portal blood–unfiltered*)

   ○ 6. Branch of bile duct

○ 7. Sinusoids

The lobes of the liver are divided into thousands of functional microscopic units called **lobules**. Blood is delivered to the lobules via the liver's two sources of blood supply: the **hepatic artery**, which carries oxygen-rich blood from the heart, and the **hepatic portal vein**, carrying nutrients from the digestive system.

Hepatocytes

(Enlarged view of the liver lobule)

○   1. White blood cell
A – Portal triad
    ○   2. Hepatic artery
    ○   3. Branch of portal vein
    ○   4. Branch of bile duct
○   5. Bile canaliculi
○   6. Sinusoid
○   7. Red blood cell
○   8. Kupffer cell
       (reticuloendothelial cell)
○   9. Hepatocyte
○   10. Fat storing cell

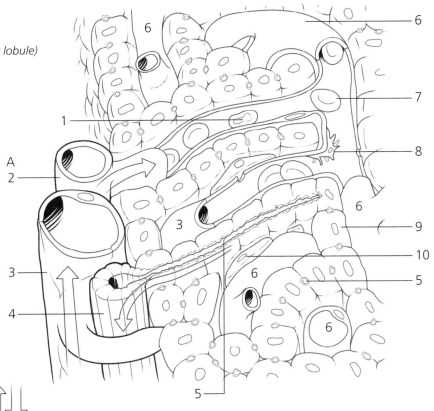

PHYSIOLOGY:
Liver lobule function

○   1. Branch of bile duct
○   2. Branch of portal vein
○   3. Hepatic artery
–   4. To the inferior vena cava
○   5. Central vein
○   6. Liver lobule
–   7. Bile collects in the common bile duct
–   8. Deoxygenated and processed blood returning to the heart
–   9. Oxygenated blood from the heart
–   10. Blood from the digestive system

The four lobes of the liver are divided into thousands of functional microscopic units called **lobules**. Blood is delivered to the lobules via the liver's two sources of blood supply: the hepatic artery, which carries oxygen-rich blood from the heart, and the hepatic portal vein, carrying nutrients from the digestive system.

The DIGESTIVE System

(Frontal view – sections removed for clarity)

The portal system

- — 1. To heart
- ○ 2. Inferior vena cava *(cut)*
- — 3. Liver
- ○ 4. Hepatic portal vein
- ○ 5. Gastric vein
- — 6. Small intestine *(cut)*
- ○ 7. Superior mesenteric vein
- — 8. Large intestine *(cut)*
- ○ 9. Inferior mesenteric vein
- — 10. Intestinal veins
- — 11. Esophagus *(cut)*
- — 12. Stomach *(cut)*
- ○ 13. Spleen
- ○ 14. Left gastroepiploic vein
- ○ 15. Splenic vein
- ○ 16. Right colic vein
- — 17. Rectum

11.13

(Frontal view – sections removed for clarity)

Bile production

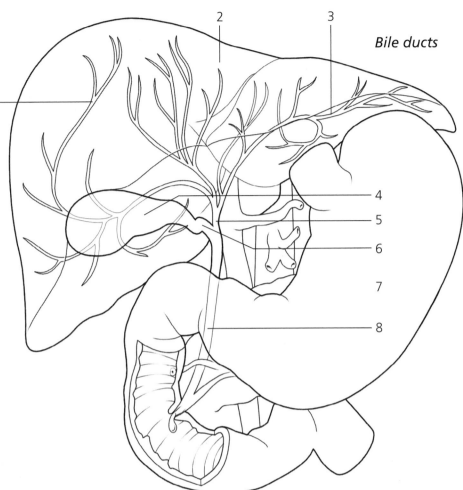

Bile ducts

○ 1. Right hepatic duct
○ 2. Liver
○ 3. Left hepatic duct
○ 4. Gallbladder
○ 5. Common hepatic duct
– 6. Cystic duct
– 7. Stomach
○ 8. Common bile duct

Coloring guide suggestion
*When coloring, use same
color to indicate similar parts*

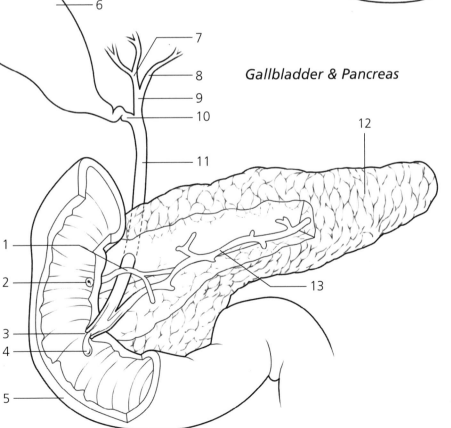

Gallbladder & Pancreas

○ 1. Accessory pancreatic duct
– 2. Minor duodenal papilla
– 3. Major duodenal papilla
○ 4. Bile and pancreatic juice
– 5. Duodenum
○ 6. Gallbladder
○ 7. Right hepatic duct
○ 8. Left hepatic duct
○ 9. Common hepatic duct
– 10. Cystic duct
○ 11. Common bile duct
○ 12. Pancreas
○ 13. Main pancreatic duct

11.14

ANATOMY & PHYSIOLOGY COLORING BOOK

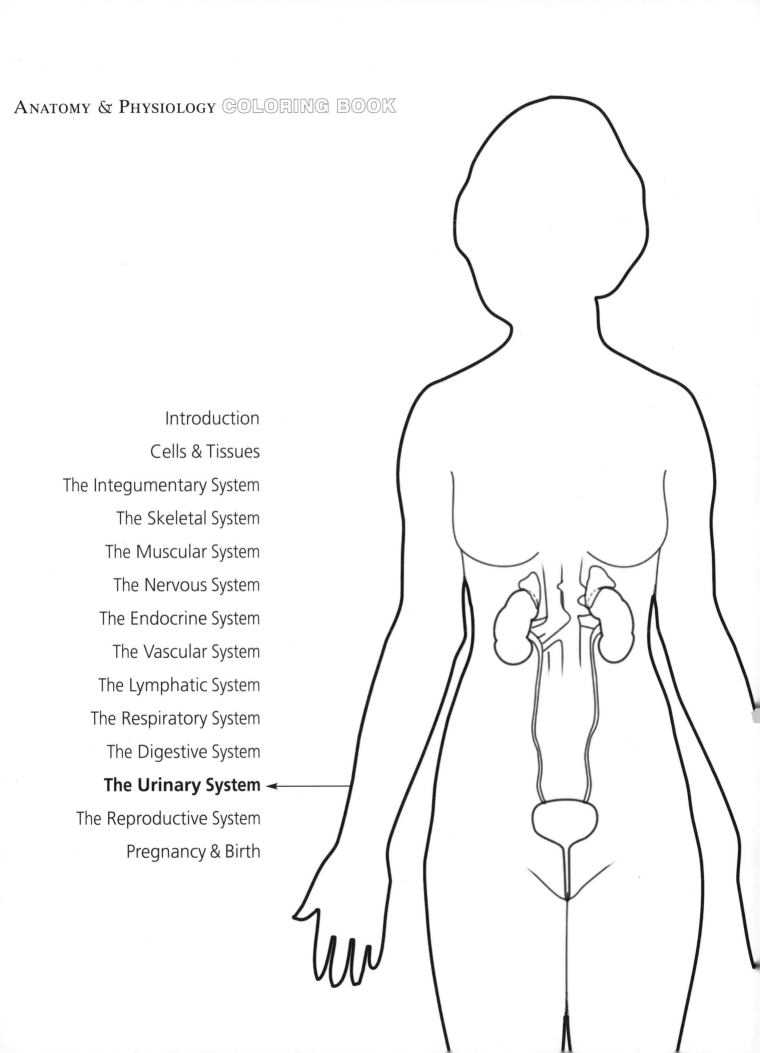

The URINARY System

System overview

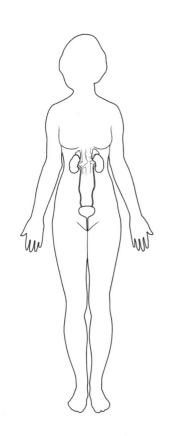

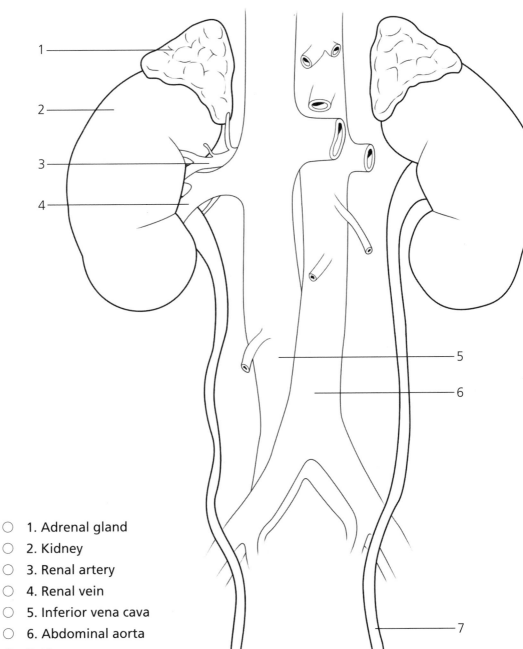

- ○ 1. Adrenal gland
- ○ 2. Kidney
- ○ 3. Renal artery
- ○ 4. Renal vein
- ○ 5. Inferior vena cava
- ○ 6. Abdominal aorta
- ○ 7. Ureter
- ○ 8. Urinary bladder

The urinary system is responsible for three major functions in the body: removing metabolic wastes, maintaining normal water volume, and controlling acid-base (pH) balance in the bloodstream. A complex three-step process of filtration, reabsorption and secretion removes metabolic wastes, allows important substances such as glucose and water to be passed back into the blood, and eliminates toxins such as drugs and ammonia.

The URINARY System

System overview: Male

(Diagrammatic view)

○ 1. Kidney
○ 2. Ureter
○ 3. Urinary bladder
○ 4. Urethra
○ 5. Prostate gland

The URINARY System

System overview: Male

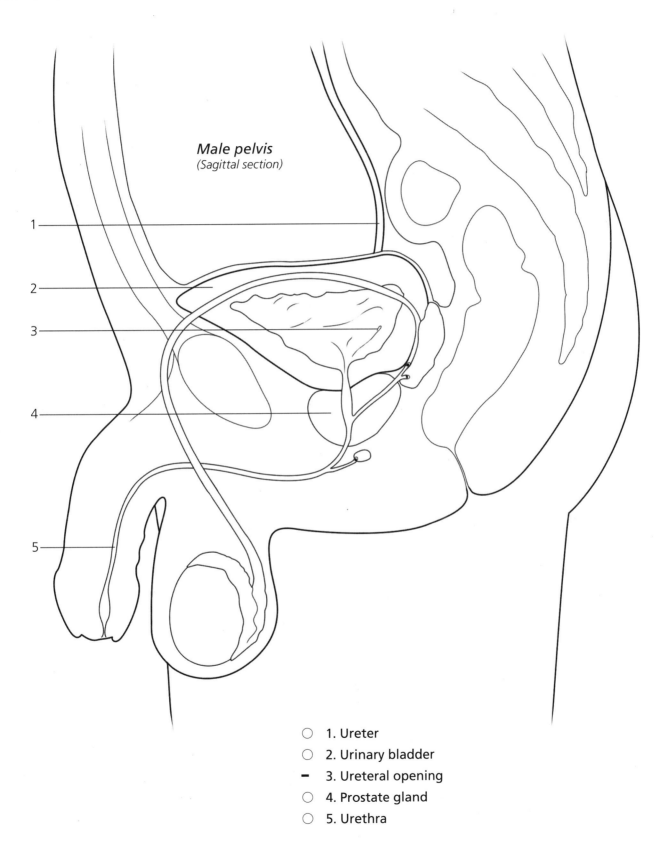

Male pelvis
(Sagittal section)

1
2
3
4
5

○ 1. Ureter
○ 2. Urinary bladder
— 3. Ureteral opening
○ 4. Prostate gland
○ 5. Urethra

The URINARY System

System overview: Female

(Diagrammatic view)

○ 1. Kidney
○ 2. Ureter
○ 3. Urinary bladder
○ 4. Urethra
○ 5. Uterus
○ 6. Vagina

The URINARY System

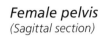

System overview: Female

Female pelvis
(Sagittal section)

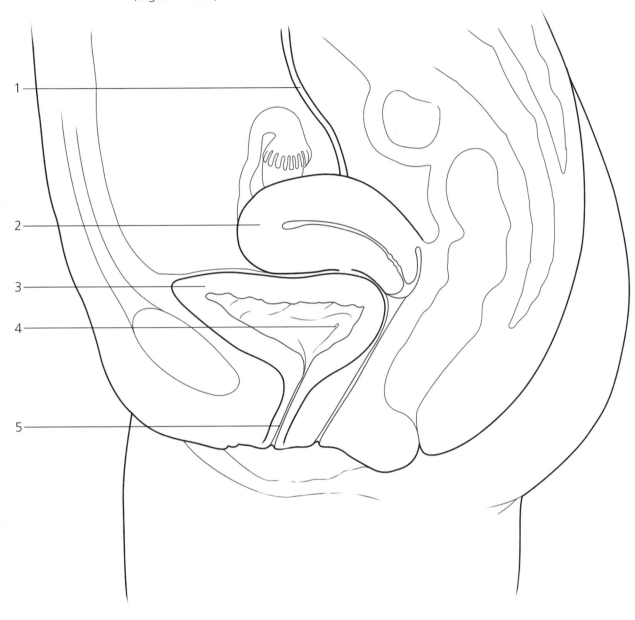

- ○ 1. Ureter
- ○ 2. Uterus
- ○ 3. Urinary bladder
- — 4. Ureteral opening
- ○ 5. Urethra

The URINARY System

Segments of the kidney

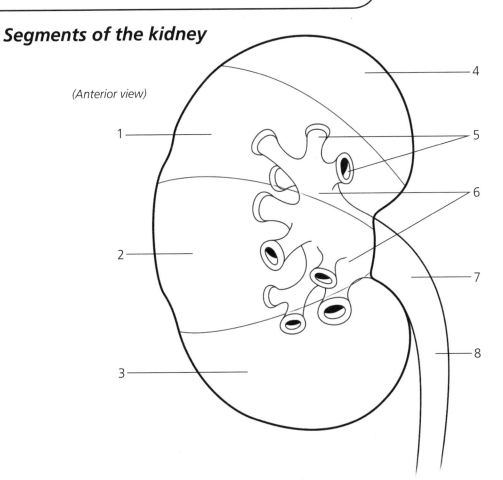

(Anterior view)

- ○ 1. Anterosuperior segment
- ○ 2. Anteroinferior segment
- ○ 3. Inferior segment
- ○ 4. Apical segment
- ○ 5. Minor calyces
- ○ 6. Major calyces
- − 7. Renal pelvis
- ○ 8. Ureter

Coloring guide suggestion
*When coloring, use same
color to indicate similar parts*

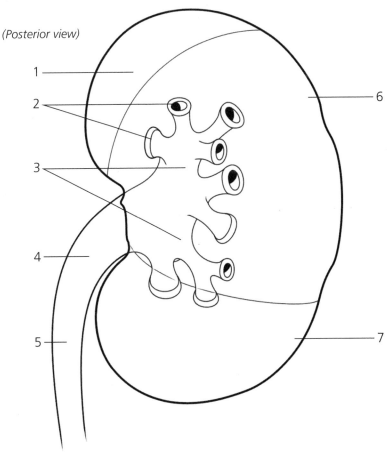

(Posterior view)

- ○ 1. Apical segment
- ○ 2. Minor calyces
- ○ 3. Major calyces
- − 4. Renal pelvis
- ○ 5. Ureter
- ○ 6. Posterior segment
- ○ 7. Inferior segment

12.6

The URINARY System

The kidney

(Frontal view – sections removed for clarity)

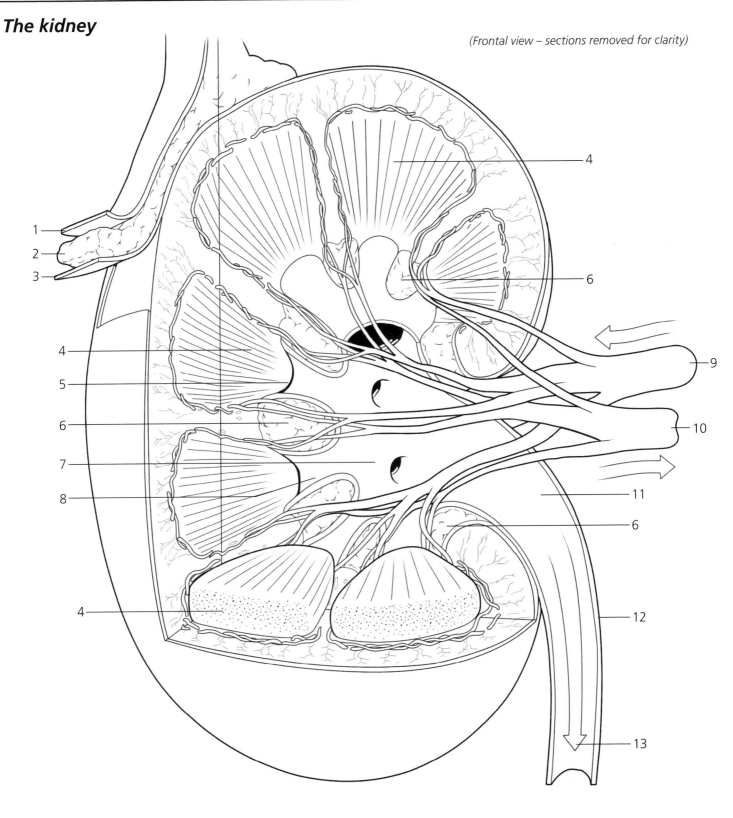

○ 1. Renal fascia   ○ 6. Fat in renal sinus   – 11. Renal pelvis

○ 2. Perirenal fat   – 7. Major calyx   ○ 12. Ureter

○ 3. Fibrous capsule   – 8. Minor calyx   ○ 13. Flow of urine

○ 4. Renal pyramid   ○ 9. Renal artery

– 5. Renal papilla   ○ 10. Renal vein

The URINARY System

The kidney

(Frontal view – sections removed for clarity)

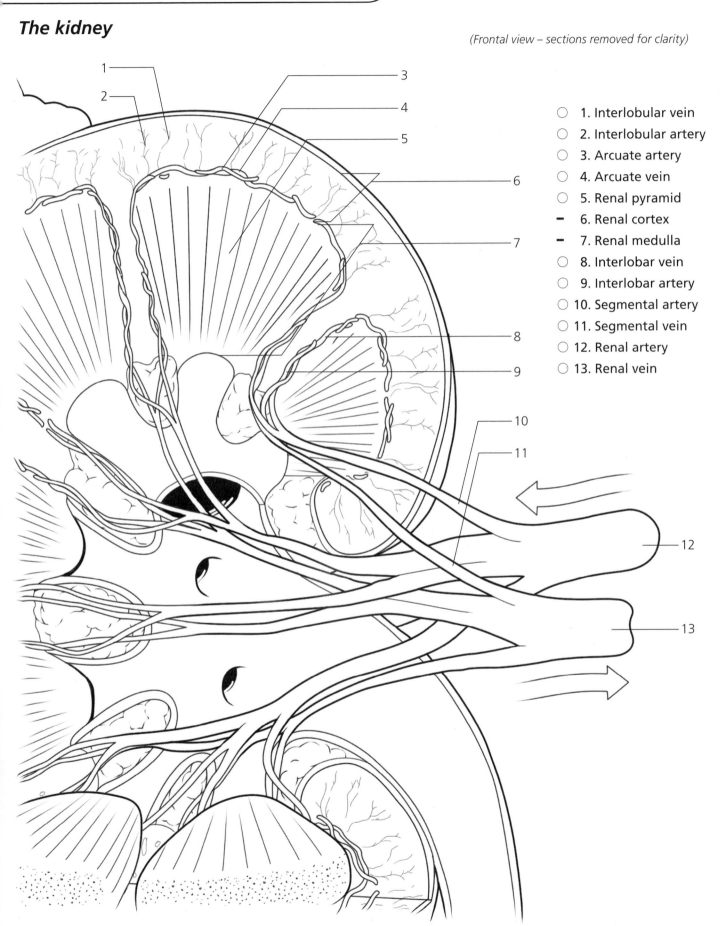

- ○ 1. Interlobular vein
- ○ 2. Interlobular artery
- ○ 3. Arcuate artery
- ○ 4. Arcuate vein
- ○ 5. Renal pyramid
- – 6. Renal cortex
- – 7. Renal medulla
- ○ 8. Interlobar vein
- ○ 9. Interlobar artery
- ○ 10. Segmental artery
- ○ 11. Segmental vein
- ○ 12. Renal artery
- ○ 13. Renal vein

The URINARY System

The nephron

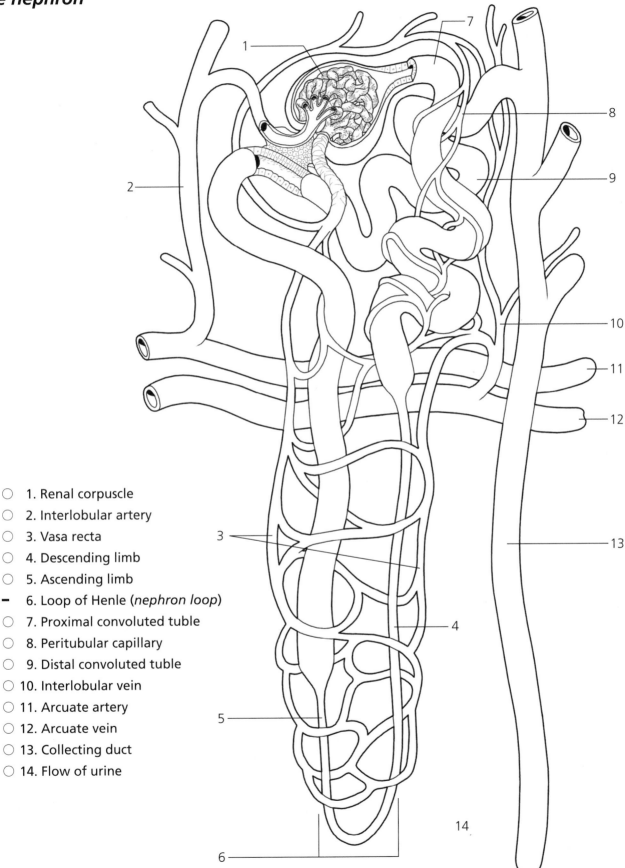

○ 1. Renal corpuscle
○ 2. Interlobular artery
○ 3. Vasa recta
○ 4. Descending limb
○ 5. Ascending limb
– 6. Loop of Henle (*nephron loop*)
○ 7. Proximal convoluted tuble
○ 8. Peritubular capillary
○ 9. Distal convoluted tuble
○ 10. Interlobular vein
○ 11. Arcuate artery
○ 12. Arcuate vein
○ 13. Collecting duct
○ 14. Flow of urine

The glomerulus

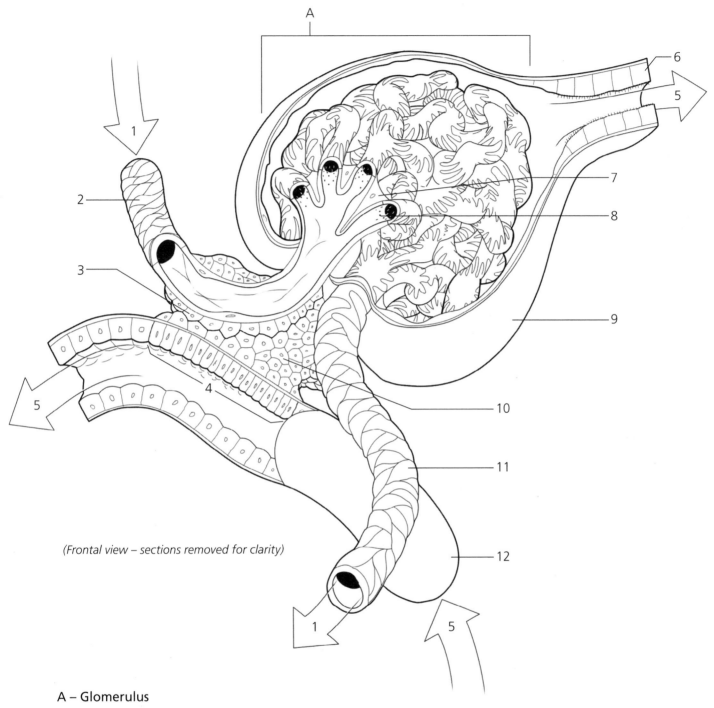

(Frontal view – sections removed for clarity)

A – Glomerulus

○ 1. Blood flow
○ 2. Afferent arteriole
○ 3. Juxtaglomerular cells
○ 4. Macula densa
○ 5. Filtrate flow
– 6. Proximal convoluted tuble (*PCT*)

○ 7. Mesangial cell
– 8. Fenestration (*pore*)
○ 9. Glomerular capsule
○ 10. Extra glomerular mesangial cell
○ 11. Efferent arteriole
– 12. Distal convoluted tuble (*DCT*)

The URINARY System

Glomerular capillary

PHYSIOLOGY:
Glomerular filtration

(Diagrammatic view)

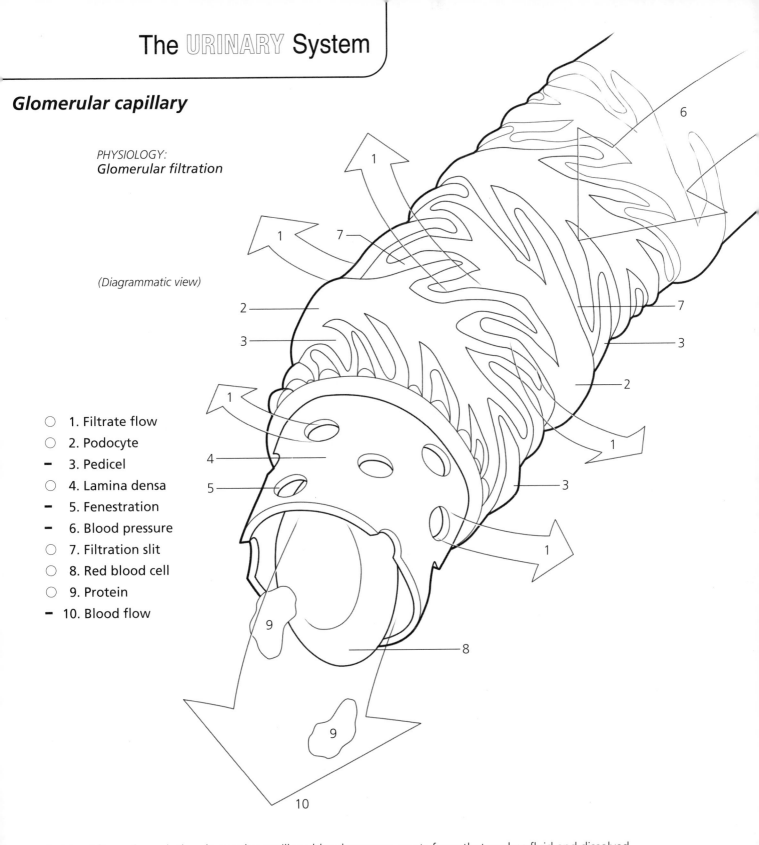

○ 1. Filtrate flow
○ 2. Podocyte
− 3. Pedicel
○ 4. Lamina densa
− 5. Fenestration
− 6. Blood pressure
○ 7. Filtration slit
○ 8. Red blood cell
○ 9. Protein
− 10. Blood flow

As blood flows through the glomerular capillary, blood pressure exerts force that pushes fluid and dissolved substances through the filtration apparatus. The pores in the fenestrated capillary are large enough to allow plasma and solutes to diffuse, but too small for blood cells to pass. The basement membrane (**lamina densa**) is thicker and more dense than a typical basement membrane, allowing smaller proteins and nutrients to pass.

The outer surface of the basement membrane is surrounded with **podocytes**, specialized cells with long processes, or **pedicels**, that wrap around the capillary membrane. The pedicels are separated by very narrow gaps called **filtration slits**. The combination of high fluid pressure, selectively permeable membranes and large filtration surface areas allows a large volume of fluid to be filtered.

Filtrate formation in the nephron

PHYSIOLOGY:
Filtrate formation in the nephron

(Diagrammatic view)

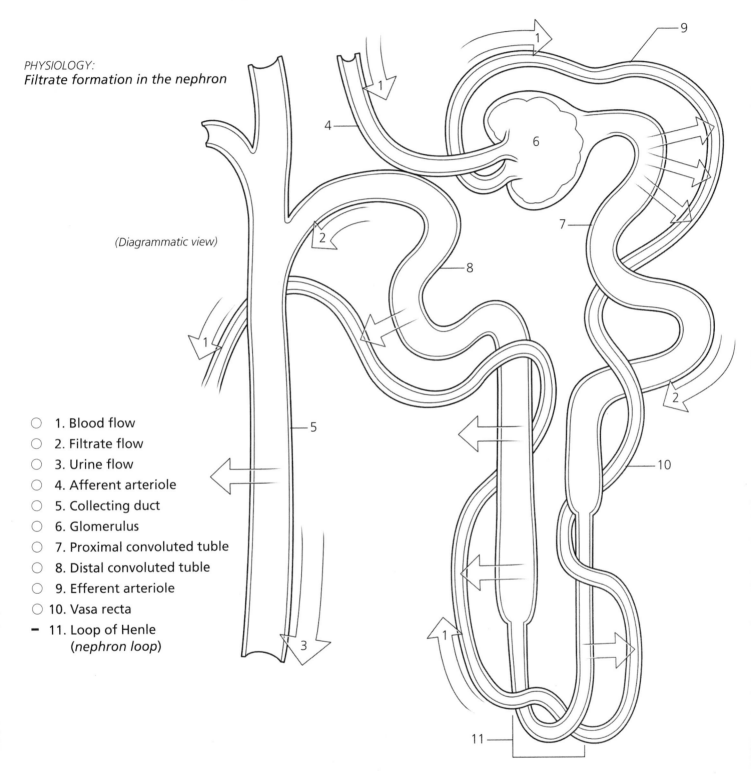

○ 1. Blood flow
○ 2. Filtrate flow
○ 3. Urine flow
○ 4. Afferent arteriole
○ 5. Collecting duct
○ 6. Glomerulus
○ 7. Proximal convoluted tuble
○ 8. Distal convoluted tuble
○ 9. Efferent arteriole
○ 10. Vasa recta
— 11. Loop of Henle
   (*nephron loop*)

Urine production begins when blood enters the nephrons via the afferent arterioles. After a complex process of reabsorption and secretion along the renal tubule, concentrated urine containing water and wastes such as sodium and **urea** (a by-product of toxic ammonia products formed in the liver) leaves the collecting ducts. The kidneys process an average of 200 quarts of blood daily, eventually excreting only about 2 quarts of extra water and waste products as urine.

Filtrate formation in the nephron – step 1

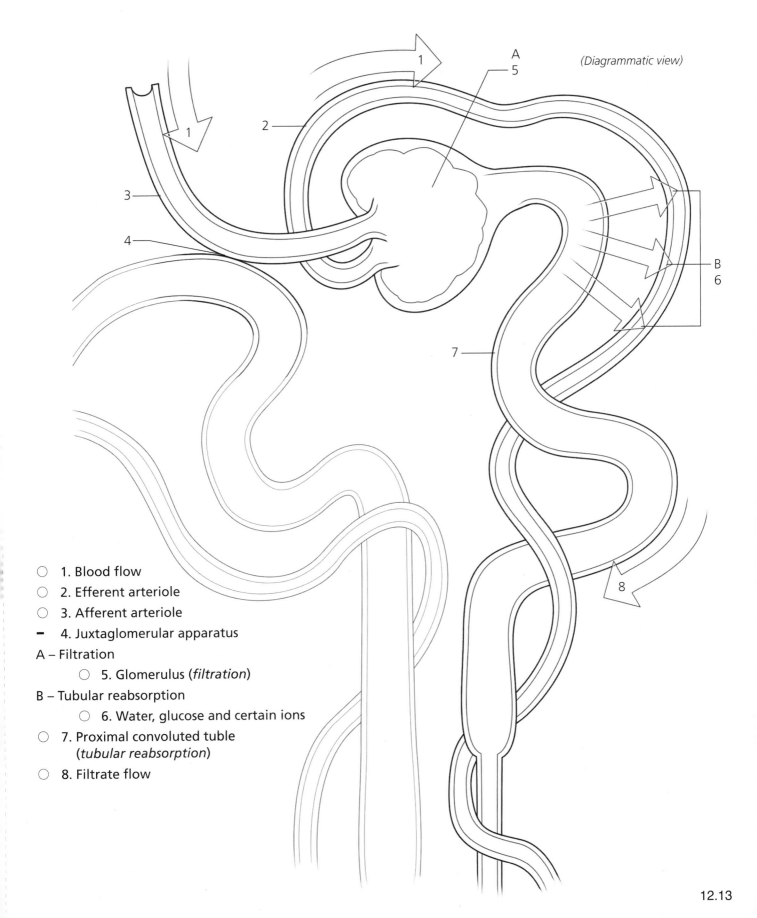

(Diagrammatic view)

○ 1. Blood flow
○ 2. Efferent arteriole
○ 3. Afferent arteriole
– 4. Juxtaglomerular apparatus
A – Filtration
        ○ 5. Glomerulus (*filtration*)
B – Tubular reabsorption
        ○ 6. Water, glucose and certain ions
○ 7. Proximal convoluted tuble
        (*tubular reabsorption*)
○ 8. Filtrate flow

The URINARY System

Filtrate formation in the nephron – step 2

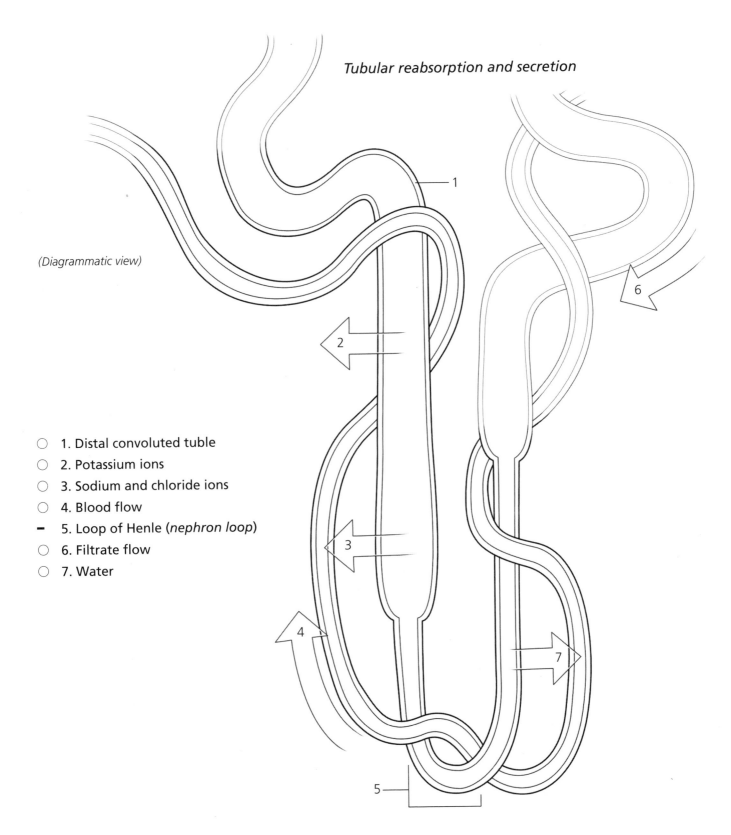

Tubular reabsorption and secretion

(Diagrammatic view)

○ 1. Distal convoluted tuble
○ 2. Potassium ions
○ 3. Sodium and chloride ions
○ 4. Blood flow
– 5. Loop of Henle (nephron loop)
○ 6. Filtrate flow
○ 7. Water

Filtrate formation in the nephron – step 3

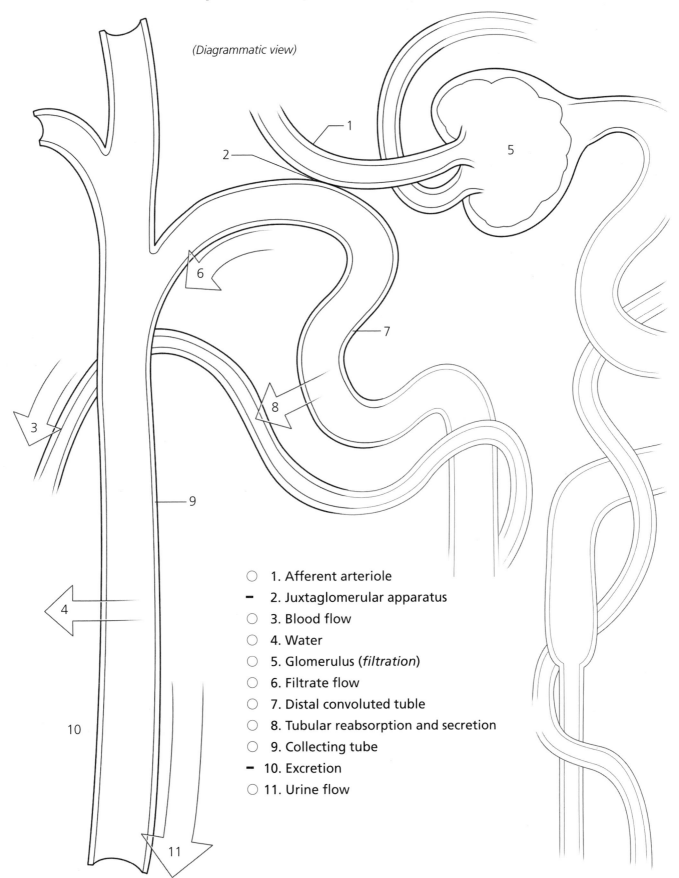

(Diagrammatic view)

○ 1. Afferent arteriole
− 2. Juxtaglomerular apparatus
○ 3. Blood flow
○ 4. Water
○ 5. Glomerulus (*filtration*)
○ 6. Filtrate flow
○ 7. Distal convoluted tuble
○ 8. Tubular reabsorption and secretion
○ 9. Collecting tube
− 10. Excretion
○ 11. Urine flow

ANATOMY & PHYSIOLOGY COLORING BOOK

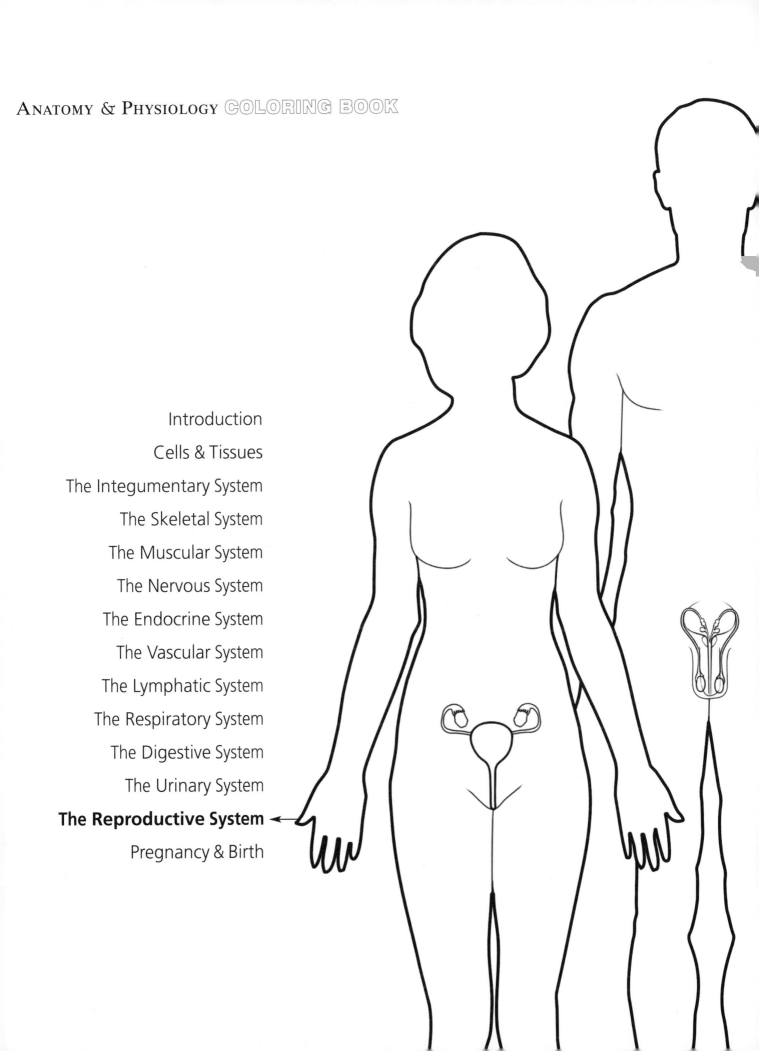

The REPRODUCTIVE System

System overview

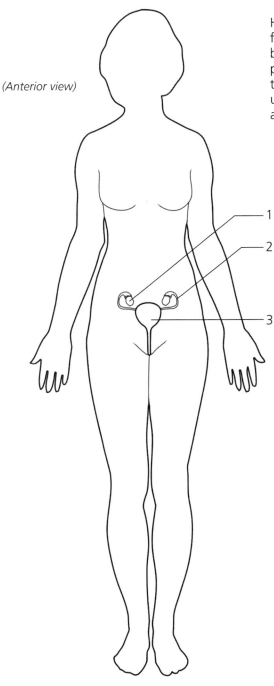

(Anterior view)

Humans reproduce by sexual reproduction involving male and female reproductive cells called **gametes**. Reproduction is regulated by hormones produced by the gonads, the hypothalamus and the pituitary gland. Fertilization involves the introduction of semen into the vagina. The sperm travels through the female reproductive tract until it encounters an **oocyte**, a female immature gamete. Union of a sperm and the oocyte (**fertilization**) can then take place.

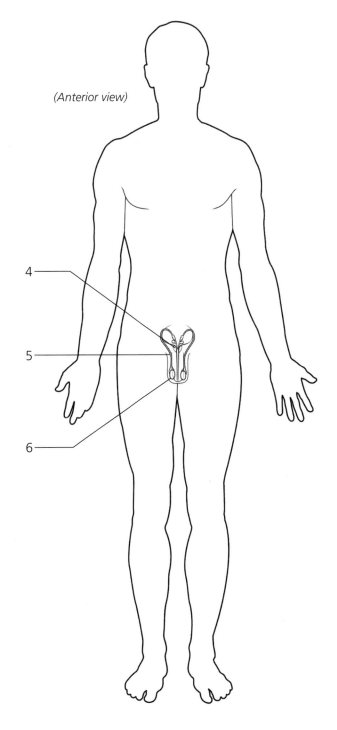

(Anterior view)

○ 1. Ovary
○ 2. Uterine tube
○ 3. Uterus
○ 4. Prostate gland
○ 5. Ductus deferens
○ 6. Testis

The REPRODUCTIVE System

System overview: Male

Zones of the prostate

A – Seminal vesicle
B – Ductus deferens
C – Testicle
D – Urethra

(Diagrammatic view)

- 1. Bladder
○ 2. Ampulla of vans deferens
○ 3. Seminal vesicle
- 4. Prostate gland
○ 5. Central zone
○ 6. Peripheral zone
○ 7. Transition zone
○ 8. Anterior zone
○ 9. Ejaculatory duct
- 10. Urethra

○ 1. Urinary bladder
○ 2. Ampulla of vans deferens
○ 3. Seminal vesicle
○ 4. Prostate gland
- 5. Penis
○ 6. Ductus deferens
○ 7. Urethra
○ 8. Testis

13.2

Spermiogenesis

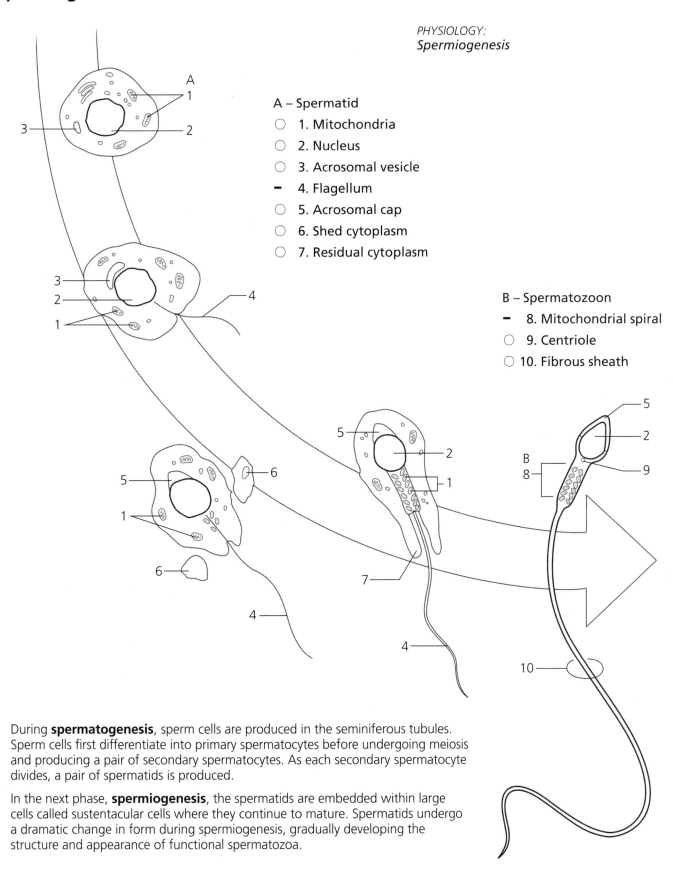

PHYSIOLOGY:
Spermiogenesis

A – Spermatid
- ○ 1. Mitochondria
- ○ 2. Nucleus
- ○ 3. Acrosomal vesicle
- — 4. Flagellum
- ○ 5. Acrosomal cap
- ○ 6. Shed cytoplasm
- ○ 7. Residual cytoplasm

B – Spermatozoon
- — 8. Mitochondrial spiral
- ○ 9. Centriole
- ○ 10. Fibrous sheath

During **spermatogenesis**, sperm cells are produced in the seminiferous tubules. Sperm cells first differentiate into primary spermatocytes before undergoing meiosis and producing a pair of secondary spermatocytes. As each secondary spermatocyte divides, a pair of spermatids is produced.

In the next phase, **spermiogenesis**, the spermatids are embedded within large cells called sustentacular cells where they continue to mature. Spermatids undergo a dramatic change in form during spermiogenesis, gradually developing the structure and appearance of functional spermatozoa.

The REPRODUCTIVE System

Movement of spermatozoa

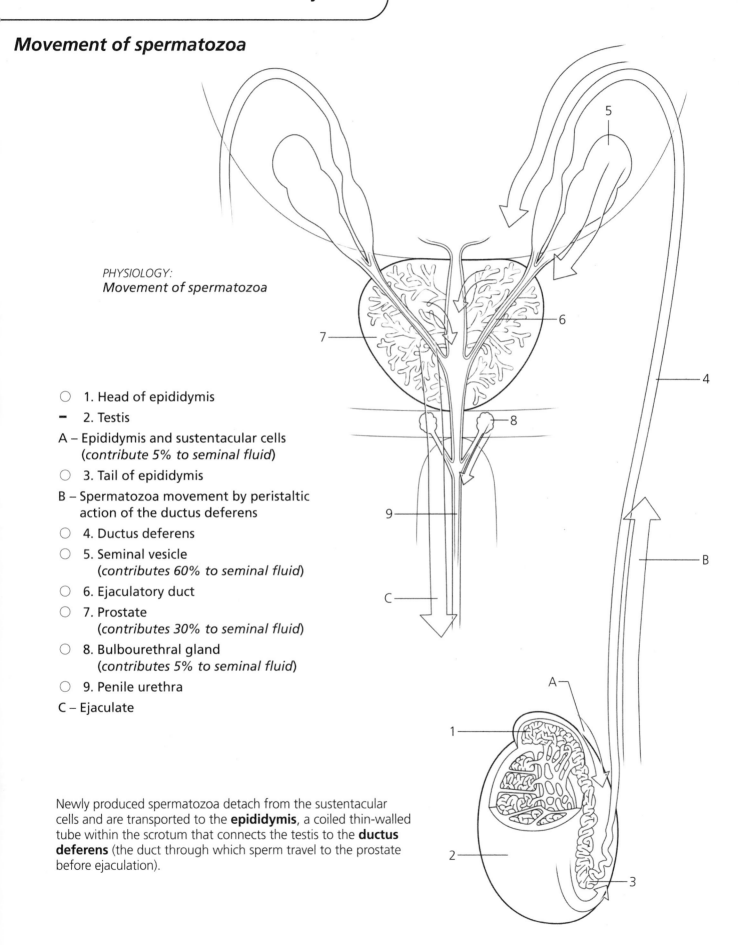

PHYSIOLOGY:
Movement of spermatozoa

○ 1. Head of epididymis

− 2. Testis

A – Epididymis and sustentacular cells
(*contribute 5% to seminal fluid*)

○ 3. Tail of epididymis

B – Spermatozoa movement by peristaltic
action of the ductus deferens

○ 4. Ductus deferens

○ 5. Seminal vesicle
(*contributes 60% to seminal fluid*)

○ 6. Ejaculatory duct

○ 7. Prostate
(*contributes 30% to seminal fluid*)

○ 8. Bulbourethral gland
(*contributes 5% to seminal fluid*)

○ 9. Penile urethra

C – Ejaculate

Newly produced spermatozoa detach from the sustentacular
cells and are transported to the **epididymis**, a coiled thin-walled
tube within the scrotum that connects the testis to the **ductus
deferens** (the duct through which sperm travel to the prostate
before ejaculation).

The REPRODUCTIVE System

System overview: Female

(Diagrammatic view)

A – Ovary
B – Uterine tube
C – Uterus
D – Vagina

- ○ 1. Uterine tube
- ○ 2. Ovary
- ○ 3. Uterus
- – 4. Cervix
- ○ 5. Urinary bladder
- – 6. Vagina

(Frontal view – sections removed for clarity)

- – 1. Fundus of uterus
- – 2. Body of uterus
- ○ 3. Ovarian ligament
- ○ 4. Ovary
- ○ 5. Uterosacral ligament
- ○ 6. Cervical canal
- ○ 7. Uterine tube
- ○ 8. Uterine cavity
- ○ 9. Endometrium
- ○ 10. Myometrium
- ○ 11. Perimetrium
- ○ 12. Cervix
- ○ 13. Vagina

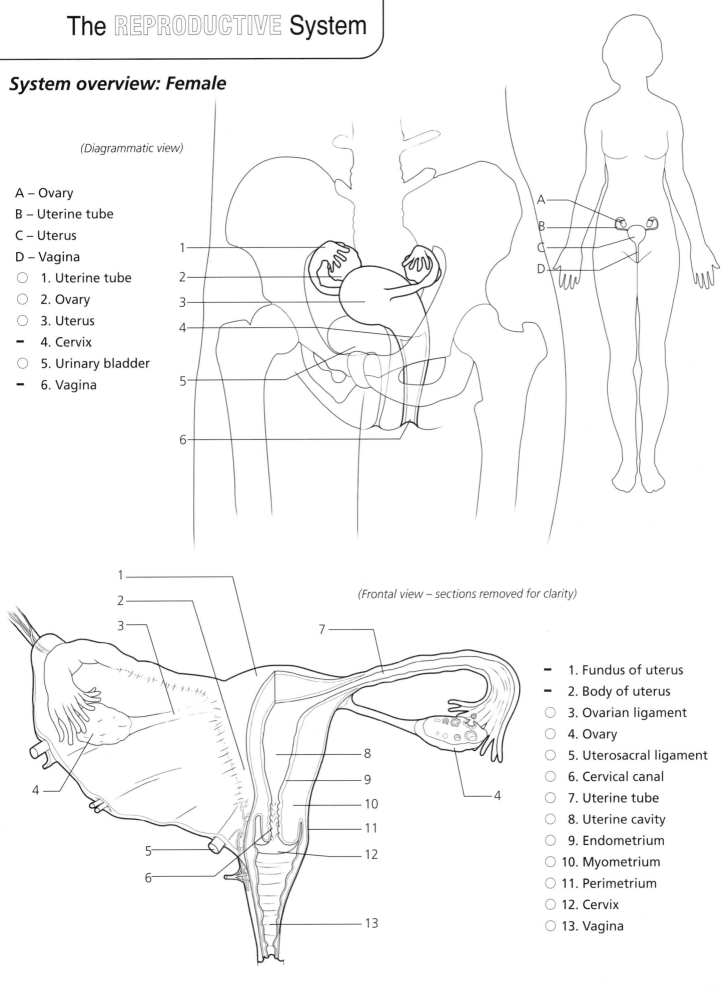

The REPRODUCTIVE System

Ovulation

Uterine tube and ovary
(Coronal section)

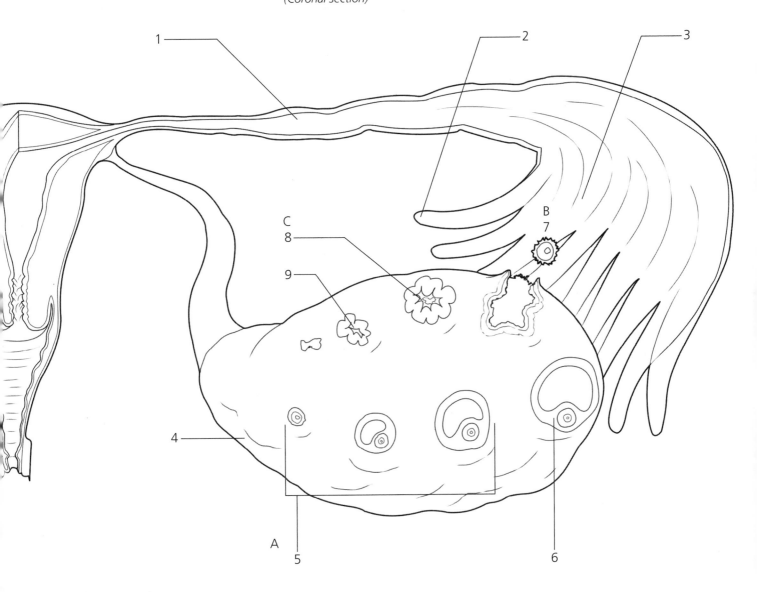

○ 1. Uterine tube
– 2. Fimbriae of uterine tube
○ 3. Infundibulum of uterine tube
○ 4. Ovary
A – Follicular phase
    ○ 5. Developing follicle
    ○ 6. Mature follicle
B – Follicular phase
    ○ 7. Ovulation
C – Luteal phase
    ○ 8. Corpus luteum
    ○ 9. Corpus albicans

Ovulation is the release of a single mature ovum from one of the ovaries, which is triggered by a sudden rise in the blood level of the gonadotrophin hormone LH. The ovum travels down the uterine tube and enters the uterine cavity. An unfertilized ovum passes out of the body through the vagina.

Ovulation normally occurs around day 14 of the menstrual cycle.

The REPRODUCTIVE System

The menstrual cycle

○ 1. Endometrium
○ 2. Vagina
○ 3. Uterine tube
○ 4. Uterus
○ 5. Ovary
– 6. Ovulation
○ 7. Menstruation

PHYSIOLOGY:
The menstrual cycle

(Diagrammatic view)

The menstrual cycle refers to the sequence of events that occurs in the **endometrium**, the cell layer lining the uterus. This cycle normally lasts for approximately 28 days. Its purpose is to prepare the uterus for possible pregnancy.

If fertilization does not occur, decreasing estrogen and progesterone levels initiate menstruation and the cycle begins again.

Ovulation phases

Days 0   14   26   0

Ovarian hormones

○ 1. Ovaries
○ 2. Uterus
○ 3. Ovulation
– 4. Follicular Phase
– 5. Luteal Phase
○ 6. Estrogen
○ 7. Progesterone

The menstrual cycle is governed by the endocrine system. During the first two weeks, the pituitary gland releases follicle stimulating hormone (FSH) to stimulate egg growth in the ovary. Ripening eggs produce estrogen, causing thickening of the uterine lining. About 14 days into the cycle, levels of luteinizing hormone (LH) increase, triggering the release of a ripened egg (follicle).

13.7

The REPRODUCTIVE System

Gametes

A – Oocyte (*egg cell*) at ovulation
- ○ 1. Zona pellucida
- ○ 2. Ovum
- ○ 3. Corona radiata
- ○ 4. Polar body

B – Spermatozoon
- ○ 5. Acrosomal cap
- ○ 6. Nucleus
- ○ 7. Centriole
- − 8. Mitochondrial spiral
- ○ 9. Fibrous sheath

A

1
2
3

4

(Coronal view)

B
5
6
7
8
9

Coloring guide suggestion
*When coloring, use same
color to indicate similar parts*

PHYSIOLOGY:
Fertilization

A

1

2
3
4

(Coronal view)

5

A – Path is cleared by enzymes
released from the acrosome
- ○ 1. Spermatozoon
- ○ 2. Ovum
- ○ 3. Zona pellucida
- ○ 4. Corona radiata
- ○ 5. Polar body

The upper portion of the uterine tube is the usual place for fertilization. Millions of sperm travel through the female reproductive tract, although only about 100 make it all the way to the egg. When a sperm meets the **corona radiata**, cells surrounding the egg, the acrosome of the sperm ruptures, releasing enzymes that allow the sperm to reach the egg surface.

13.8

The REPRODUCTIVE System

Fertilization

Acrosomal reaction

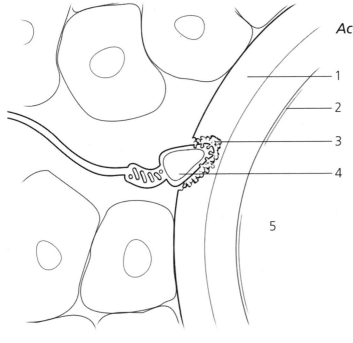

- ○ 1. Zona pellucida
- ○ 2. Ovum plasma membrane
- ○ 3. Enzymes
- ○ 4. Sperm cell nucleus
- — 5. Ovum cytoplasm

> **Coloring guide suggestion**
> *When coloring, use same
> color to indicate similar parts*

Fusion of plasma membranes

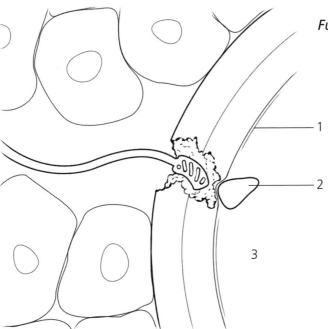

- ○ 1. Plasma membrane
- ○ 2. Sperm cell nucleus
- — 3. Ovum cytoplasm

The sperm travels through a path made by the digestive action of the enzymes released from the acrosome. When the cell membranes of the egg and sperm come in contact, the membranes fuse, and the sperm nucleus and associated material move into the egg. Other sperm are prevented from entering by a chemical change in the zona pellucida.

The egg's nuclear membrane disappears, the chromosomes of the egg and sperm combine, and a fertilized egg, or zygote, is created.

13.9

Sex determination

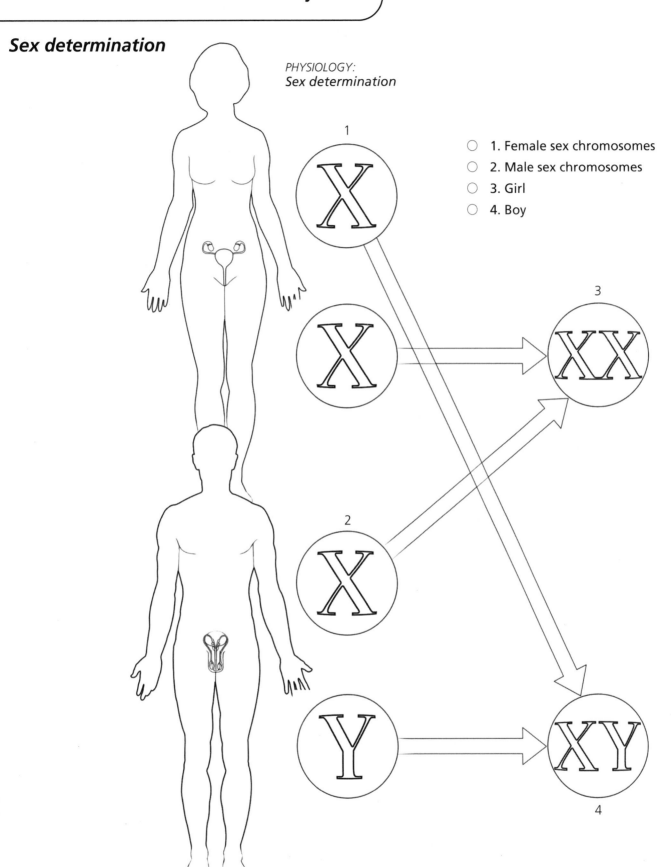

PHYSIOLOGY:
Sex determination

○ 1. Female sex chromosomes
○ 2. Male sex chromosomes
○ 3. Girl
○ 4. Boy

Each parent contributes one sex chromosome. The mother always contributes an
X sex chromosome, while the father contributes either an X or a Y sex chromosome.
An XX combination produces a girl, while a boy has an XY combination.

ANATOMY & PHYSIOLOGY COLORING BOOK

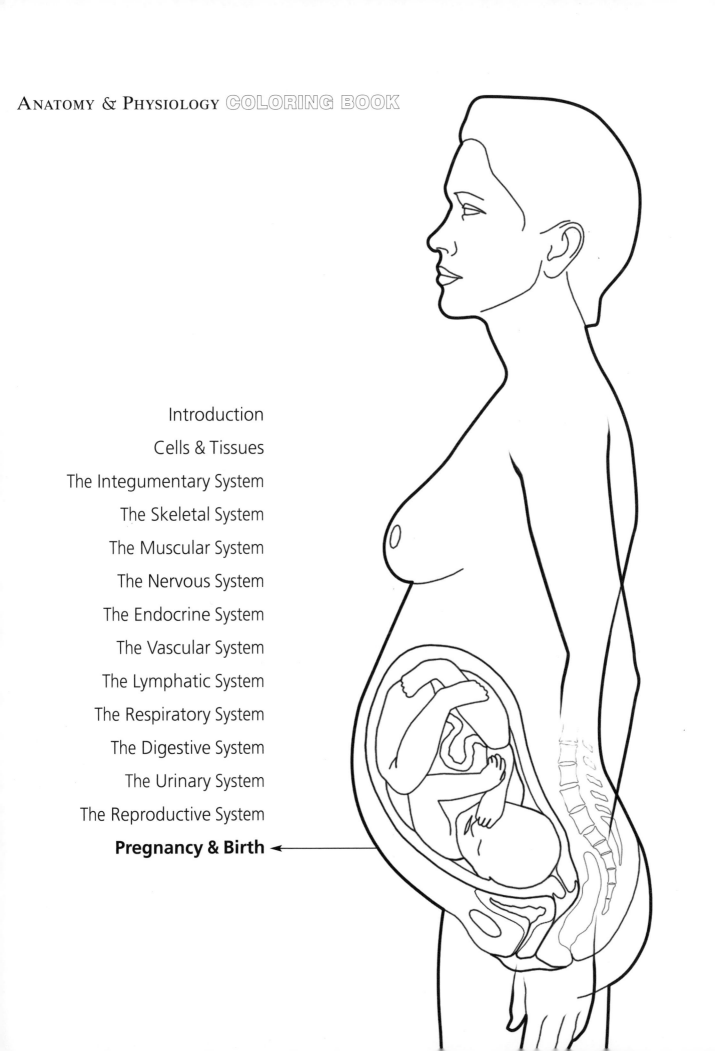

System overview

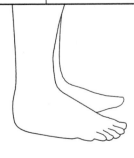

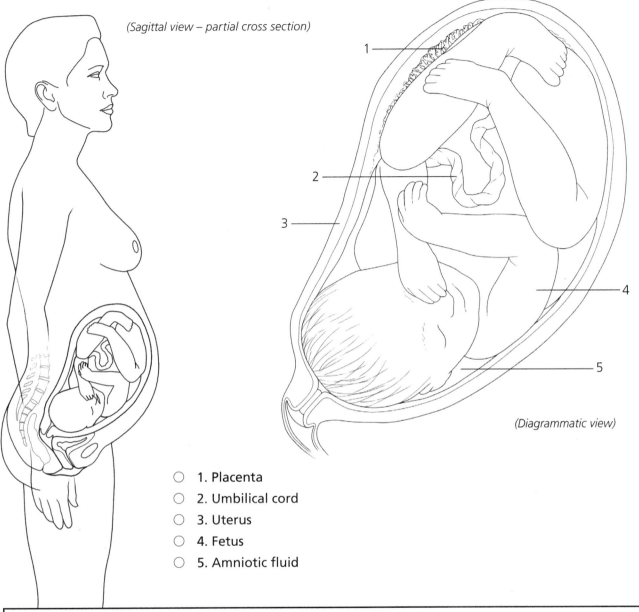

(Sagittal view – partial cross section)

(Diagrammatic view)

○ 1. Placenta
○ 2. Umbilical cord
○ 3. Uterus
○ 4. Fetus
○ 5. Amniotic fluid

Pregnancy Weeks, Months, Trimesters																																									
Week	1	2	3	4	5	6	7	8	9	10	11	12	13	14	15	16	17	18	19	20	21	22	23	24	25	26	27	28	29	30	31	32	33	34	35	36	37	38	39	40	41	42
Month	1				2				3				4				5				6				7				8				9				10						
Trimester	1												2												3													4				

Pregnancy lasts approximately 40 weeks from the first day of the last menstrual period. The earliest sign that a fertilized egg has successfully implanted and pregnancy has begun is often a missed menstrual period, which is confirmed by either a urine or a blood test and physical examination. As the fetus develops, the mother's body undergoes many physiologic changes to support its expanding nutritional and growth needs. The three primary stages of fetal development are called **trimesters**.

Ovulation

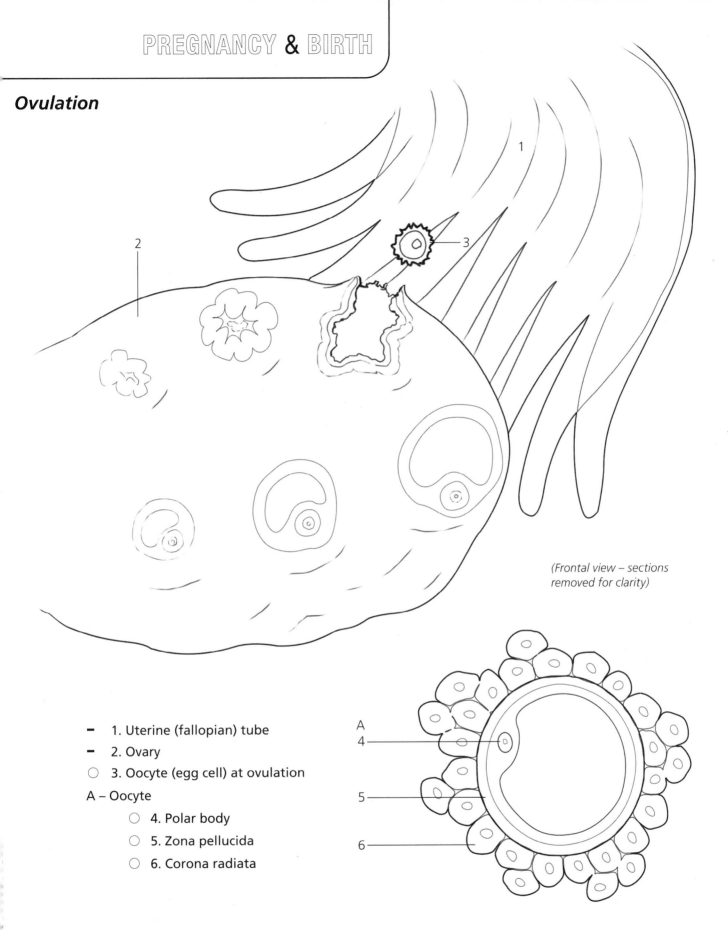

(Frontal view – sections removed for clarity)

− 1. Uterine (fallopian) tube

− 2. Ovary

○ 3. Oocyte (egg cell) at ovulation

A – Oocyte

    ○ 4. Polar body

    ○ 5. Zona pellucida

    ○ 6. Corona radiata

Ovulation occurs at approximately day 14 of the menstrual cycle, when increased levels of luteinizing hormone signal the release of a single mature ovum (egg) from one of the ovaries. Once released, the egg passes through the uterine (fallopian) tube to the uterus.

Fertilization

A – Fertilization and activation of oocyte
- ○ 1. Spermatozoa
- ○ 2. Fertilizing sperm cell membrane fuses with the egg cell membrane
- ○ 3. Ovum
- – 4. Uterine tube
- – 5. Ovary

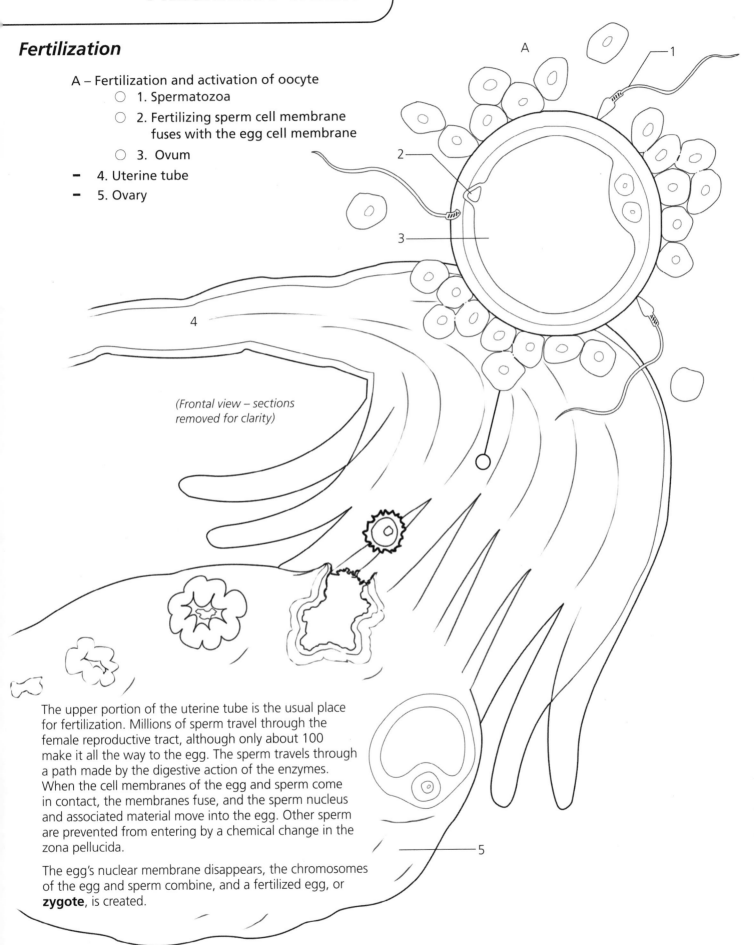

A

(Frontal view – sections removed for clarity)

The upper portion of the uterine tube is the usual place for fertilization. Millions of sperm travel through the female reproductive tract, although only about 100 make it all the way to the egg. The sperm travels through a path made by the digestive action of the enzymes. When the cell membranes of the egg and sperm come in contact, the membranes fuse, and the sperm nucleus and associated material move into the egg. Other sperm are prevented from entering by a chemical change in the zona pellucida.

The egg's nuclear membrane disappears, the chromosomes of the egg and sperm combine, and a fertilized egg, or **zygote**, is created.

14.3

Zygote

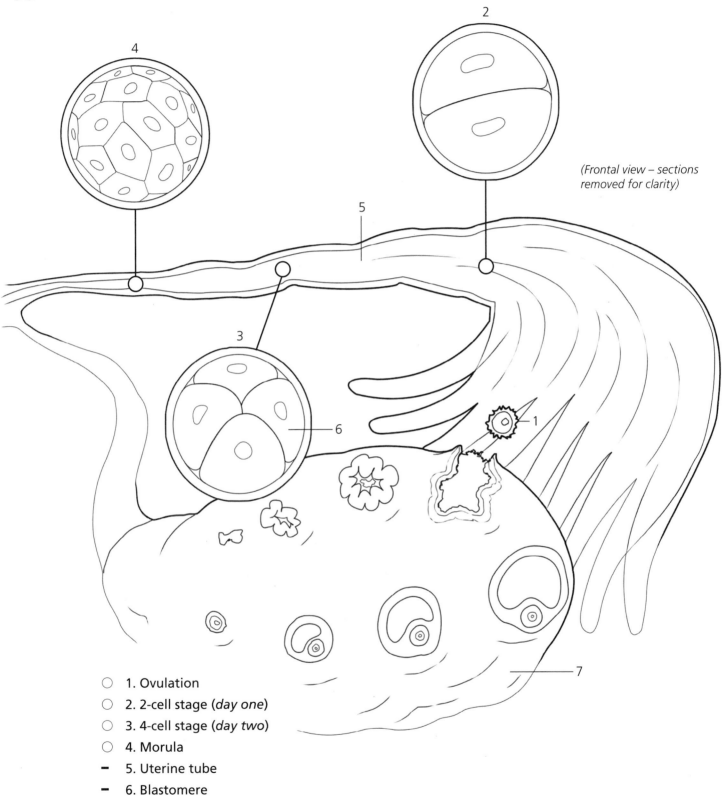

(Frontal view – sections removed for clarity)

○ 1. Ovulation
○ 2. 2-cell stage (*day one*)
○ 3. 4-cell stage (*day two*)
○ 4. Morula
– 5. Uterine tube
– 6. Blastomere
– 7. Ovary

Zygote

Fertilized egg

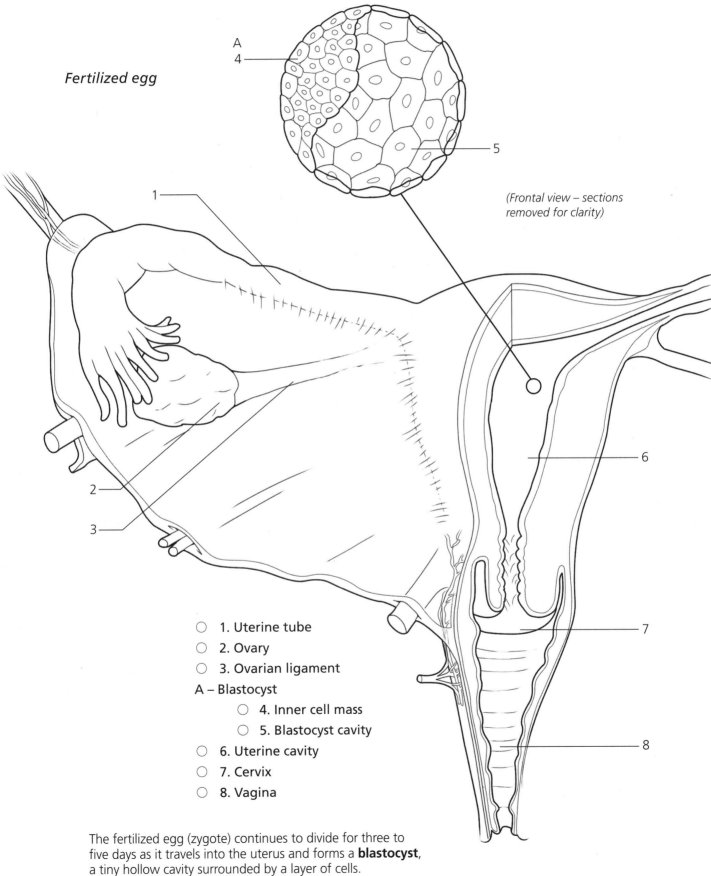

A
4

5

(Frontal view – sections removed for clarity)

○ 1. Uterine tube
○ 2. Ovary
○ 3. Ovarian ligament
A – Blastocyst
    ○ 4. Inner cell mass
    ○ 5. Blastocyst cavity
○ 6. Uterine cavity
○ 7. Cervix
○ 8. Vagina

The fertilized egg (zygote) continues to divide for three to five days as it travels into the uterus and forms a **blastocyst**, a tiny hollow cavity surrounded by a layer of cells.

Implantation

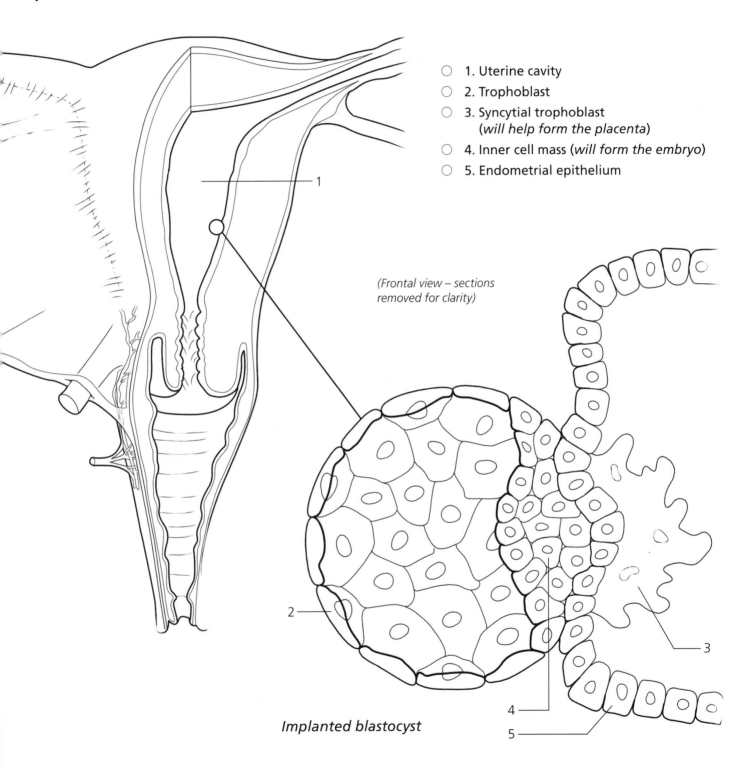

○ 1. Uterine cavity

○ 2. Trophoblast

○ 3. Syncytial trophoblast
(*will help form the placenta*)

○ 4. Inner cell mass (*will form the embryo*)

○ 5. Endometrial epithelium

*(Frontal view – sections
removed for clarity)*

Implanted blastocyst

Five to eight days after fertilization, the blastocyst begins to implant in the lining of the uterine wall (**endometrium**). New layers of cells eventually develop into the placenta, and an amniotic sac filled with fluid encloses the blastocyst, which is now called an **embryo**.

14.6

Coloring guide suggestion
*When coloring, use same
color to indicate similar parts*

Blastocysts

Single mass blastocyst

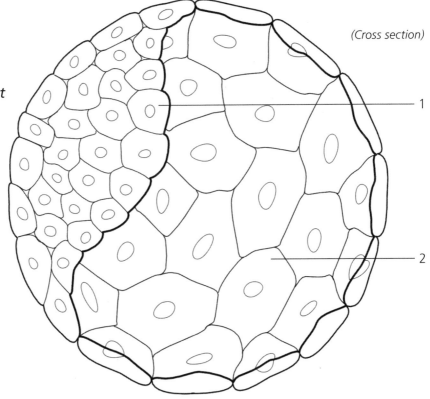

(Cross section)

1

2

○ 1. Inner cell mass
○ 2. Blastocyst cavity

A – Monozygotic (*identical*) twin development

 ○ 2. Blastocyst cavity
 ○ 3. Two inner cell masses

Two mass blastocyst

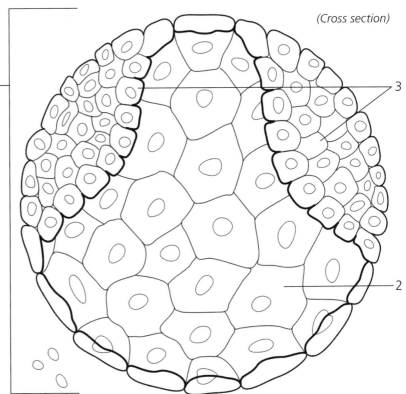

(Cross section)

A

3

2

Multiple births

In a multiple pregnancy, more than one fetus develops in the uterus. Twins are the most common type of multiple pregnancy, and are estimated to occur in one of every 80 pregnancies. Multiple pregnancies can occur naturally or as a result of infertility drugs that allow more than one mature ovum to be released and subsequently fertilized.

There are two kinds of multiple siblings. If multiple separate eggs are released and fertilized, the babies will be fraternal siblings. When a single fertilized egg separates into two embryos after it has begun to divide, the siblings will be identical.

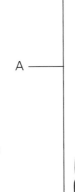

Pregnancy

The role of the placenta

During implantation, the outer cells of the blastocyst become embedded in the uterus, contributing to the development of the placenta. The **placenta** is a specialized organ with numerous small projections (**villi**) extending into the blood vessels of the uterine wall. As the mother's blood flows into the spaces surrounding the villi, nutrients, oxygen and antibodies are exchanged with the blood of the fetus through a thin membrane. Waste products from the fetus flow back into the mother's body through the same membrane. The placenta continues to grow throughout the pregnancy and weighs about one pound at birth.

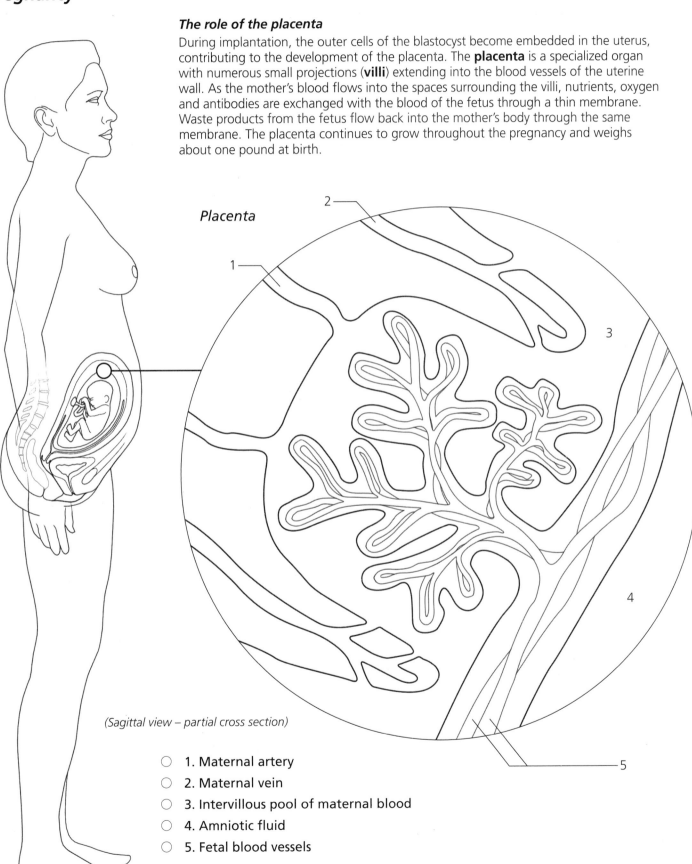

Placenta

(Sagittal view – partial cross section)

○ 1. Maternal artery

○ 2. Maternal vein

○ 3. Intervillous pool of maternal blood

○ 4. Amniotic fluid

○ 5. Fetal blood vessels

14.8

Pregnancy
First trimester

(Side view – sections removed for clarity)

A – Uterus

B – Fetus

C – Bladder

○ 1. Placenta

○ 2. Umbilical cord

○ 3. Yolk sac

○ 4. Mucus plug

○ 5. Cervix

○ 6. Vagina

○ 7. Fetus

○ 8. Amniotic fluid

– 9. Uterine cavity

First trimester
During the first three months, the embryo undergoes rapid transformation. Primitive germ cell layers evolve into the body's major organs and structures, including a neural tube (early spinal cord), bones, muscles, lungs, kidneys and liver. The heart begins beating between the third and fouth weeks.

Pregnancy
Second trimester

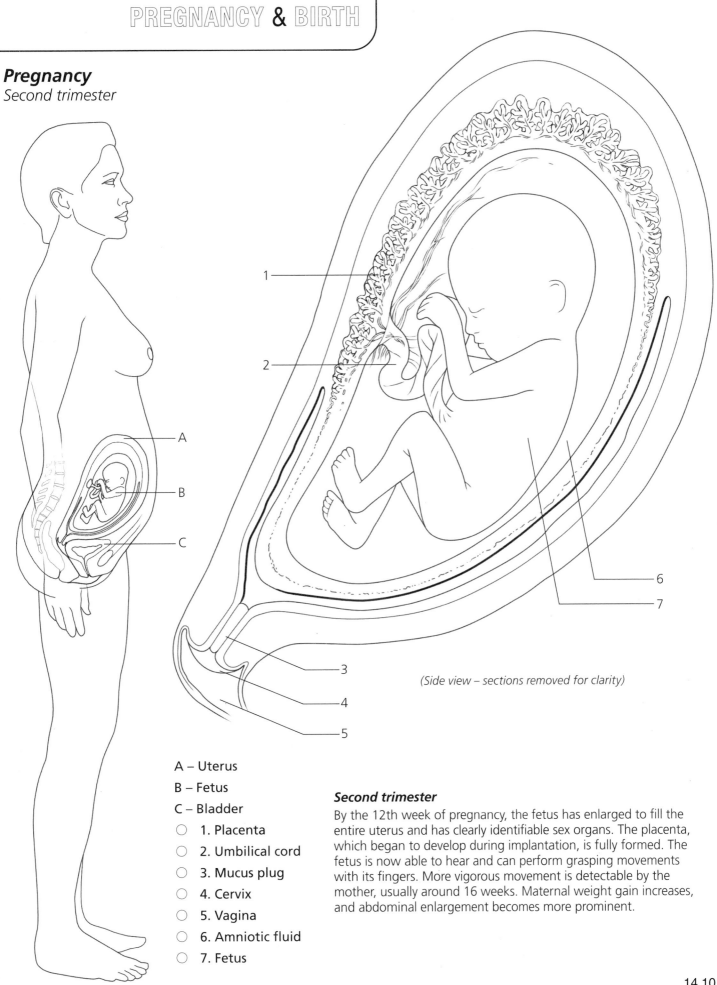

1
2
6
7
3
4
5

(Side view – sections removed for clarity)

A
B
C

A – Uterus

B – Fetus

C – Bladder

○ 1. Placenta

○ 2. Umbilical cord

○ 3. Mucus plug

○ 4. Cervix

○ 5. Vagina

○ 6. Amniotic fluid

○ 7. Fetus

Second trimester
By the 12th week of pregnancy, the fetus has enlarged to fill the entire uterus and has clearly identifiable sex organs. The placenta, which began to develop during implantation, is fully formed. The fetus is now able to hear and can perform grasping movements with its fingers. More vigorous movement is detectable by the mother, usually around 16 weeks. Maternal weight gain increases, and abdominal enlargement becomes more prominent.

Pregnancy
Third trimester

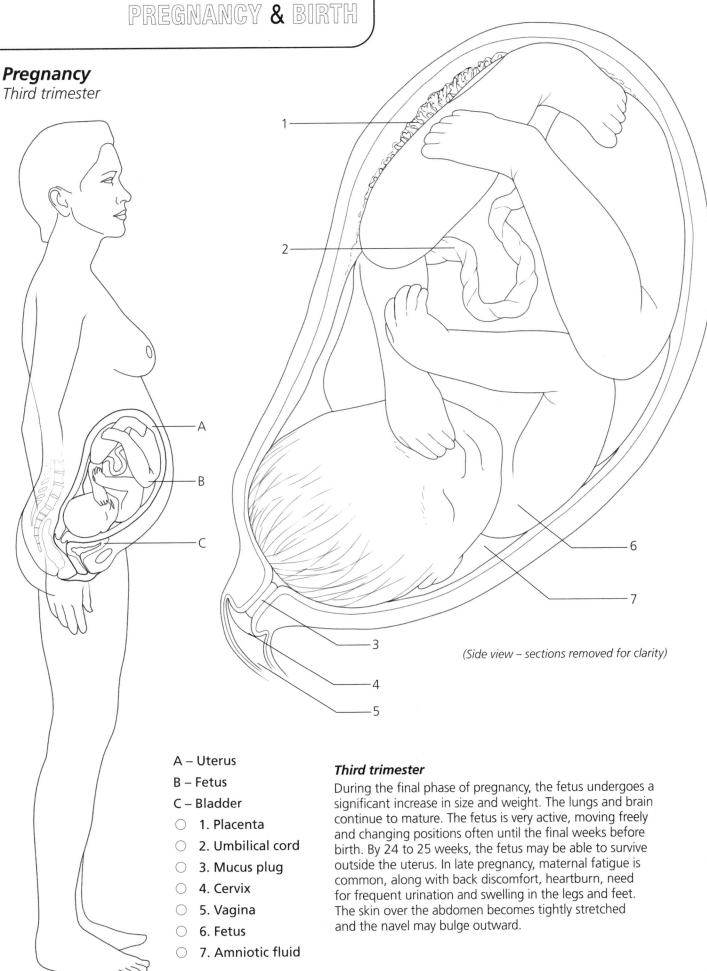

A – Uterus

B – Fetus

C – Bladder

○ 1. Placenta

○ 2. Umbilical cord

○ 3. Mucus plug

○ 4. Cervix

○ 5. Vagina

○ 6. Fetus

○ 7. Amniotic fluid

(Side view – sections removed for clarity)

Third trimester

During the final phase of pregnancy, the fetus undergoes a significant increase in size and weight. The lungs and brain continue to mature. The fetus is very active, moving freely and changing positions often until the final weeks before birth. By 24 to 25 weeks, the fetus may be able to survive outside the uterus. In late pregnancy, maternal fatigue is common, along with back discomfort, heartburn, need for frequent urination and swelling in the legs and feet. The skin over the abdomen becomes tightly stretched and the navel may bulge outward.

Delivery and birth

(Diagrammatic views)

○ 1. Contractions
○ 2. Umbilical cord
– 3. Ruptured amniotic sac
– 4. Vagina (*birth canal*)
○ 5. Widening cervix
○ 6. Placenta
– 7. "Crowning"
○ 8. Uterus

Birth begins with **labor**, a series of rhythmic and progressive contractions of the uterus that cause the cervix to become thin (**effaced**) and dilate. As labor progresses, the fetus is gradually pushed from the uterus through the widened cervix and into the birth canal. Labor usually begins two weeks before or after the estimated due date and lasts from six to fourteen hours.

14.12

Anatomical GLOSSARY

A

Accommodation, the ability of the eye to keep an image focused on the retina

Adrenal glands, a pair of endocrine glands that secrete steroid hormones

Agonist, a muscle that produces an action

Alveolus, pockets at the end of respiratory bronchioles

Amphiarthroses, slightly movable joints

Antagonist, a muscle that opposes an action

Antibody, a protein that binds to specific antigens to promote their removal or destruction

Arachnoid granulations, collections of villi or projections providing a path for reentry of CSF into the venous system

Artery, blood vessel carrying blood away from the heart

Articulation, a joint or any location in the body where two or more bones come together

Astrocytes, a type of supporting cell in neural tissue

AV node, atrioventricular node; specialized cells that pass a stimulus to the bundle branches

Axon, a long extension of the cell membrane of the neuron

B

Basement membrane, connects epithelium and underlying connective tissue

Bile, secretion of the liver, stored in the gallbladder, used in digestion

Blastomeres, two identical cells produced by mitotic division

Blood, a type of connective tissue comprised of plasma (a liquid matrix) and formed elements (red and white blood cells, and platelets)

Bolus, a mixture of food and saliva

Bone, a type of connective tissue, with its own cells and an extracellular matrix

Bundle branches, specialized conducting cells that carry a stimulus from the AV node to the Purkinje fibers

Bursa, small fluid-filled sac that help to reduce friction between tendons and ligaments

C

Calyx, a cup-shaped drain in the kidney

Capillaries, small blood vessels connecting arteries and veins

Carotene, a yellow-orange pigment primarily evident in the stratum corneum of the skin and in subcutaneous fat

Chemoreceptors, specialized nerve cells that respond to molecules dissolved in fluid, i.e., mucus and saliva

Chewing, the mechanical action of the teeth and tongue to begin the breakdown of solid food

Chondrocytes, cartilage cells

Cilia, extensions of the cell membrane

CNS, the central nervous system, including the brain and spinal cord

Colon, the large intestine

Compact bone, relatively dense; forms the walls of bones

Concentration, the amount of a substance in a given volume or area

Condyle, a rounded projection of a bone, generally a cartilage-covered joint surface

Corona radiata, the cells surrounding an egg

Cranial meninges, three layers of tissue that keep the brain from contacting the cranial bones

Crista ampullaris, inner ear sensory hair cells that respond to rotational movement

CSF, cerebrospinal fluid; a clear, watery liquid that circulates around and within the central nervous system

D

Dendrites, fiber-like extensions of a neuron

Dermatome, a specific region monitored by a pair of spinal nerves

Dermis, the dense, middle layer of the skin

Diaphysis, the shaft of a bone

Diarthroses, the most freely movable synovial joints

Diastole, cardiac relaxation, allowing a heart chamber to fill with blood

Digestion, the breakdown of food into components small enough to be absorbed

Duodenum, the first part of the small intestine

E

Endolymph, a fluid in the membranous labyrinth in the inner ear which flows in response to movement of the head and body

Endometrium, the inner lining of the uterus

Endomysium, connective tissue fibers that separate and support muscle fiber cells

Endothelium, cells lining lymphatic and blood vesssels

Epidermis, the thin, uppermost layer of the skin

Epiglottis, a flap-like valve blocking the trachea

Epiphysis, the end part of the bone

Erythrocytes, red blood cells that transport oxygen and carbon dioxide through the vascular system

Expiration, expelling air from the lungs during a complete breath

Expiratory reserve volume, the additional amount of air that can be forcibly exhaled past a normal exhalation

F

Fascicle, a bundle of muscle fiber that makes up skeletal muscles

Filtration slits, narrow gaps separating the pedicels

Foramen, an opening in bone

Frequency, the number of cycles per second, measured in Hertz (Hz)

G

Gametes, male and female reproductive cells

Gastrointestinal tract, a muscular tube in which intake, digestion and absorption of nutrients, and elimination takes place

Glial cells, support cells found in the CNS and PNS

Glomerulus, renal corpuscle containing a capillary network

Gonads, reproductive organs that produce gametes and hormones

Gustation, the sense of taste

Gustatory cell, chemoreceptor found in the taste bud

H

Haustra, pouches along the length of the large intestine, caused by tension of the taenia coli

Hepatic portal system, venous blood vessels connecting the digestive system and the liver

Hepatocyte, a liver cell

Hormones, internal chemical messengers that regulate and control functions within the body

Hypodermis, the subcutaneous layer of the skin

Hypothalamus, a region of the brain with numerous functions, including control of the autonomic nervous system

I

Inflammation, a nonspecific defense response characterized by redness, swelling and warmth

Inspiration, taking air into the lungs during a complete breath

Inspiratory reserve volume, the additional amount of air that can be forcibly inhaled past a normal inhalation

Intensity, relates to the amplitude of sound waves, measured in decibels

Interneurons, nerve cells that coordinate and integrate sensory inputs and motor outputs

K

Keratin, a fibrous, tough protein found in hair, nails and outer protective skin surfaces

Keratinocyte, keratin-producing cells found throughout the integumentary system

L

Langerhans cells, cells in the skin and digestive tract; important in immune protection

Larynx, cartilaginous cylinder protecting the glottis; also known as the voice box

Leukocytes, white blood cells that are part of the immune system

Ligament, connective fibers connecting one bone to another

Lumen, the space within an internal passageway, such as a duct

Lymph, a fluid formed from excess fluid from the body's tissues

Lymph nodes, small organs that monitor lymph composition

M

Macula, sensory patch containing tiny hairs that move in response to gravity

Medullary cavity, the center of a bone that contains bone marrow

Melanin, a brown pigment produced by melanocytes

Melanocyte, skin cell that produces melanin, responsible for skin color

Melanosome, a vesicle that transfers melanin to keratinocytes

Meninges, protective membranes (dura, arachnoid and pia mater) covering the CNS

Merkel cells, skin cells involved in sensation

Metaphysis, a narrow zone separating the bone shaft (diaphysis) from the end of the bone (epiphysis)

Microvilli, extensions of the cell membrane used to increase surface area

Motor neuron, relays signals from the CNS to effector (muscle and gland) cells

Mucosa, a mucous membrane

Mucus, a secretion used for lubrication

Muscle fibers, elongated cells with the ability to contract along their length

Myelin sheath, a layer of lipid-like Schwann cells surrounding the axon

Myelin sheath gaps, the spaces between Schwann cells along an axon

Myocardium, muscle tissue of the heart

Myofibrils, cylindrical structures responsible for muscle contractions

Myofilaments, make up myofibrils; composed of two proteins called actin and myosin

N

Negative feedback, a type of regulation where an increase in the output decreases the input

Nephrons, functional units of the kidney that filter blood

Neurotransmitters, chemical messengers that carry impulses across the synaptic cleft

Nociceptors, a sensory neuron that responds to stimuli and sends signals to the brain

O

Olfaction, the detection of odors

Oocyte, a female immature gamete

Optic chiasma, the crossing point of the two optic nerves

Os coxa, i.e., the hip bone, consists of three separate bones: the ilium, pubis and ischium

Ossification, a mixture of osteoid and collagen fibers that is hardened by deposits of a mineral composed of calcium and phosphates

Osteoblasts, cells that secrete the organic parts of the matrix

Osteoclasts, multinucleate cells that dissolve bone matrix

Osteocytes, mature cells responsible for maintaining bone matrix

Osteoid, the organic part of the matrix

Osteoprogenitor, cells that divide to produce cells that differentiate into osteoblasts

Ovary, one of a pair of female reproductive glands

P

Pathogens, agents that cause disease

Pedicel, long process of a podocyte that wraps around a glomerular capillary

Perimysium, connective tissue sheath separating muscle fascicles

Periosteum, a layer of fibers and cells covering the outer surface of bone

Peristalsis, a series of muscle contractions

Pharynx, the throat; shared by the respiratory and digestive systems

Photoreceptors, specialized neurons that convert light into nerve impulses

PNS, peripheral nervous system, consisting of the cranial and spinal nerves and the autonomic nervous system

Podocytes, specialized cells that surround the glomerular capillaries

Positive feedback, a type of regulation where an increase in the output increases the input

Proprioceptors, slowly-adapting mechanoreceptors that monitor joint position and muscle tension

Pulmonary system, refers to the organs of the body that cycle oxygen and carbon dioxide into and out of the lungs

Purkinje fibers, specialized cells that convey a stimulus from the bundle branches to contractile cells in the ventricles

R

Refraction, bending of light as it passes from one medium to another, as through the lens

Renal cortex, the outer region of the kidney containing the nephrons

Renal medulla, the inner region of the kidney containing the renal pyramids and calyces

Renal pyramid, cone-shaped structure that transports urine to the calyces

Renal sinus, a central chamber that connects directly to the ureter

Residual volume, the air that remains in the lungs after exhaling

Retina, the innermost tunic, or layer of the eye

Rugae, folds in the stomach lining

S

Saccule, membranous sac in the inner ear; monitors linear acceleration

Saliva, a secretion of the salivary glands

Sarcomere, repeating units of two proteins called actin and myosin

Scrotum, a saclike structure that protects the testes

Segmentation, process of ringlike contractions that churn and mix waste material, but do not move the material along

Seminiferous tubules, tightly coiled structures where sperm formation takes place

Sensory neurons, communicate information from sensory receptors to the CNS

Sensory receptors, highly specialized nerve cells that help us detect light, temperature and other kinds of energy

Sesamoid bone, a bone that forms in a tendon over a joint

Sinus, a chamber or hollow space; a large dilated vessel for blood or lymph

Spicules, small struts in bone that eventually interconnect, forming spongy bone

Spinal cord, a long, fragile structure composed of nerves that transmit signals between the brain and body, enabling movement and sensation

Spleen, largest lymphatic organ; part of the immune system; stores and recycles red blood cells

Spongy bone, forms the inner bone; made of interconnected struts

Suture, a type of synarthroses (immovable joint)

Synaptic cleft, a tiny gap between a neuron and another cell

Synaptic knob, an axon terminal of a neuron

Synarthroses, immovable joints

Systole, cardiac contraction ejecting blood into another heart chamber or into arteries

T

Teniae coli, three smooth muscle bands running the length of the colon

Tastants, substances that produce taste

Tendon, connects muscles to bone, skin or another muscle

Testis, one of a pair of male reproductive glands (pl. testes)

Testosterone, primary male hormone produced by the testes

Tidal volume, the amount of air breathed in and out during normal respiration

Tonsils, lymphatic nodules located in the pharynx

Trabeculae, struts and thin plates in spongy bone

Trachea, the windpipe; an airway connecting the larynx to the primary bronchi

Transduce, to convert various types of energy into signals understood by the nervous system

U

Urine, a fluid containing dissolved substances; excreted by the kidneys

Utricle, membranous sac in the inner ear; monitors linear acceleration

V

Vagina, a muscular tube extending from the external genital organs to the cervix

Valve, structure allowing one-way flow of liquid

Vasoconstriction, contraction of blood vessels triggered by various substances

Vasodilation, expansion of blood vessels triggered by various substances

Vein, blood vessel carrying blood toward the heart

Visual field, the part of the external world that is projected onto the retina

Vital capacity, the combination of inspiratory reserve volume and expiratory reserve volume

Z

Zygote, a fertilized egg, created when an egg and sperm combine